Peyronie's Disease Handbook

A Practical Guide
for Living with
and Overcoming PD

Theodore R. Herazy, DC, LAc, Dipl Ac

Cornell-Sunrise Publishing, LLC

Cornell-Sunrise Publishing, LLC
1933 North Evergreen Avenue
Arlington Heights, IL 60004
info@natural-complementary-medicine.com

Library of Congress Control Number: 2007907387

ISBN: 1-4196-7843-4

Acknowledgments

This acknowledgment is given to express my sincere thanks and appreciation to my friend, Barry Farley for his inspiration and insightful guidance. He opened the storehouse of his experience while doing thousands of hours of research and counseling hundreds of men with Peyronie's disease. He gave us all the benefit of his unique perspective and sensitive understanding of this terrible condition.

I am most grateful to my very good friend, James Leahy for his kind and positive manner, his innovative thinking, and for doing the heavy-lifting of editing and proofreading this text. A retired educator, he saw through the clutter and clarified the overall content.

Most importantly I wish to thank my wife, Pat, my Florence Nightingale, whom I have known since kindergarten, for her unending support, her amazing strength of character, and for once again being my secret weapon. She did not give up on me when I made the most basic of mistakes by giving up on myself, and she inspired me to spend countless hours putting all this together. She, more than even I, is responsible for this book and the beginning of the current Alternative Medicine treatment of Peyronie's Disease.

Introduction

You have picked up a book about Peyronie's disease (PD) that, you will soon find, is different from any other that has ever been written on the subject.

What makes this book unique is that it actually offers the reader useful advice about living with PD – from routine activities, to understanding your spouse. Two different levels of information are presented in this book: techniques and strategies to cope with the mundane difficulties associated with PD, and considerable discussion about the many Alternative Medicine treatments of PD.

Treatment of PD is considered to be a part of living with this curse of a disease, because it is an ongoing process. When a person has PD a large measure of time and effort is given to studying and thinking about, wishing for, and being disappointed because of the lack of, successful treatment.

This book presents new ideas and real-world advice to incorporate into your daily routine to make life with PD less stressful, more normal, and a lot safer. This is not a book about what is not known, or what does not work, or dwelling on how distorted and impotent the penis can become. It does not help the reader to mark time until his PD is so out of control that surgery looks like a good option.

This book is positive and offers actual recommendations to make life with PD better. It offers help in areas of daily life where you might not have known you needed help, and other areas that are obviously crying out for help. Because so much is unknown and unrecognized in this health problem, and because most doctors do not like to deal with Peyronie's disease, little information filters down to the man with PD. If PD is known as the "orphan disease," then what does that make the man who has the problem? He is given little to no information about coping with this bizarre condition, because no one seems to care about it or its victims. Prior to this book there was no collection of practical tips and techniques to minimize discomfort and avoid additional injury to the penis.

The second and most important aspect of this book is a new treatment strategy for PD that is not offered in the **PDI** web site. The strategies are not only for treatment of the physical problem of PD, but also approaches and tactics for the emotional and interpersonal issues between spouse, child and parent. Peyronie's disease brings multiple layers of hardship, isolation, and pain into the lives of the men and women it touches. This book is the first to respond to these interpersonal stresses as well.

Please use these ideas and general information to decide for yourself how to live with and treat Peyronie's disease. Discuss all changes in your daily routine with your treating physician prior to making those changes. Please inform your doctor of your condition as you advance in your understanding of your problem.

Table of Contents

Chapter 1 – Living with Peyronie's Disease

Living with Peyronie's disease (PD) is not the same as studying it in medical school. As a subject, it is another interesting disease whose various facts must be understood and memorized. When you have PD, it is hell. It is unlike any other problem in the way it affects the man who has it, and the people around him. Since it is misunderstood and ignored by the medical profession, essentially no help or information is available about "living" with this problem. I can write this book because I have been living with PD for three years now; for the last year I have been totally PD-free.

Like most men who first notice any of the telltale primary signs of PD – pain during erection, a bump or nodule in the shaft of the penis, a bend or distortion of the penis that was not previously present – I immediately looked for answers and help from every source I could imagine. Like every man I have spoken to about his early phase of PD, I too was shocked to learn no clear or authoritative source of basic information is available for the PD sufferer.

Nowhere could I find information about living with or treating PD that made sense to me, or any therapy with a reasonable chance for success. Because I could not find information to help me live my life with PD, and with no source of information for sound and sensible ideas to protect me from hurting myself further, I had to create some rules for living with this secret problem. After communicating with many men who were searching for something that was not there, I found how grateful they were to learn of my own practical tips, observations, and "tricks" I used to help myself.

It was painfully apparent that there was a need to put this all together in book form. This book is intended to be that practical and helpful resource of ideas, information, tips, tricks, do's and don'ts for "living with PD."

Why This Book Is Necessary

Up until now there has been no resource of information helpful to the man with PD. There was no practical instruction in the ways necessary to lead a more normal and happy life, or help him to avoid accidentally injuring himself further during the course of the usual activities of daily living. A man with PD previously had no source of helpful tips written in simple, easy terms that could help him stop feeling like a PD victim and take control of his situation.

For the man who has just recently been told he has PD – a disease he likely had never heard of prior to that moment – it is doubtful he would think of asking simple and obvious questions: what kind of underwear to wear to avoid further problems, or what sexual positions are less likely to abuse his already injured penis? Most people, especially while grappling with such shocking news, do not think that far into a problem. Further, in today's busy medical offices, it is unlikely that any physician – least likely a urology specialist – would take the time or opportunity to talk with a PD sufferer about the unique problems he will face. A man needs to know about different methods of urinating with a penis that is severely bent like a cane, how to go about having his pants altered to avoid further injury to the penis, or non-medical treatment of Peyronie's disease.

Where does this information come from? Men do not like to talk about these things, and little contact occurs between men who have PD to discuss these important issues. Even the PD forums and discussion groups do not converse about these subjects; they are used as a place to gripe or repeat to anyone who will listen that no medical treatment exists for PD. The idea of using Alternative Medicine therapy for PD is generally foreign to these Internet groups, since they parrot traditional medical thinking almost exclusively. Since modern medical care is the usual standard used, very little transfer of positive or useful information takes place in a PD discussion group.

Thus, Peyronie's disease patients start out and remain almost totally in the dark about fundamental tactics and principles that could make life easier, less painful and less problematic. These men continue to not understand the larger issues of their health problem, and until someone points out some of these issues they remain ignorant of them. They are in that terrible state where they know so little about the problem that they lack enough information to ask the right questions. Thus a cycle is perpetuated of not knowing or understanding even the basic facts or effective strategies that are useful for a life with PD.

I have never spoken to a man who was actually doing all that he could to help his PD situation. The daily habits and strategies a man adopts or figures out for himself are often incorrect. In fact, most are doing things totally wrong or unnecessary, and by so doing are either hurting their problem further or living a substandard life that is misdirected by fear and ignorance of the real problem.

Every man I have consulted with admits, after visiting his doctor and learning he has PD, he left his doctor's office feeling totally unprepared to deal with this nightmare of a disease. All say they were never given the necessary level of explanation concerning what to do, or not do, as a Peyronie's sufferer. Men report being overwhelmed, not only by the initial news about PD, but also by this feeling of helplessness, which continues every day of their life from that point forward. It is as though a cloud of confusion and uncertainty blankets each day a man lives with Peyronie's disease.

Hopefully, if I have done my job with this book, a lot of your helplessness and hopelessness will be eased. You will receive information to put you in the most control of your personal situation since the first day you heard that terrible news.

Audience

This book is written for the wide and varied group of people who struggle with this disease – men who are first learning they have PD, men who have struggled with PD for many years, as well as the women and family members who deal with this problem though their association with this terrible condition.

This entire group can benefit from the practical and tested tactics for dealing with PD on a daily basis at many levels, presented here for the first time anywhere.

Purpose

Within these pages I offer ideas that are at once simple and complex, most primarily dealing with common activities of daily life that are impacted directly or indirectly by PD. This will be accomplished through strategies, hints and observations that are useful in avoiding further injury to the delicate tunica albuginea (too-ni-kuh al•boo-jin´e-ah) of the penis, where the dreaded scar of PD resides. Lastly, for those men who, in their confusion and concern for their own welfare, withdraw too far from living life to its fullest, this book offers suggestions for returning to previous activities without fear.

My PD Story

In mid-2002, on a date I do not remember because it seemed so unimportant at the time, my life took an abrupt and painful turn. As I was standing in the bathroom early one morning, doing what every man does first upon rising, I noticed a small bump on the left side of my penis. It startled me. I never noticed such a thing there before, and it was certainly not welcome in this sacred territory that all men guard so well.

Being a doctor for more 35 years, I quickly and casually went through the list of possibilities to explain this little pea-size bump. Wanting to comfort myself, I decided it was "only a varicose vein, yeah, that's right, just a little dilated blood vessel." This new feature was accepted easily as a harmless addition to my personal landscape. All men have a few dilated blood vessels down there, sometimes more obvious and sometimes less obvious. On this occasion I decided this was just a little temporary blood vessel dilatation that decided to show up for a few days and would soon leave me alone. Sure!

After a few weeks I quit feeling for it, because I came to accept that it might be one of those unimportant things that might always be there. I considered that it might be PD for just a brief moment, but then quickly dismissed it since I had always been a rather healthy and lucky person all my life. I did everything I could to deny the possibility that it was anything that could be as threatening as PD. How could I get PD? No injury, no family history, too healthy, too lucky. No. That was just a new little vein down there that just popped up. Nope. It couldn't be PD; it just couldn't.

Not So Lucky After All

Then several weeks later during a night time trip to the bathroom, with the usual night time erection, to my horror and absolute disgust, I found myself bent 15 degrees to the left! The truth of it all came crashing down on me. Good bye unimportant and simple varicose vein, hello Peyronie's disease. I knew all the basic data from school: no cause, no cure, variable course, variable signs and symptoms, variable everything, sometimes the scar becomes calcified, surgery the only accepted option although it often has bad side-effects, and on and on.

Immediately I told my wife what I had just discovered that night in the dark. I explained PD to her in some detail, but I knew she could not fully understand it all and how her life, too, was about to change.

My PD developed rapidly from that point forward. Within two months I had a compound curve – 35 degrees to the left, and 10 degrees up – along with a counterclockwise torque. During erection, I had a significant "bottle neck" deformity midway down, where the shaft stopped becoming erect due to three scars, the largest of which was "C" shaped and almost encircled the penis like a clamp.

During the early phase of scar development while I was showing rapid and alarming changes in the structure of the penis, I was busy reading all of the standard medical information about PD I could find. The more standard medical research studies I read the more depressed and discouraged I became about my prospects for ever being normal again.

There was never much actual pain during erection, but I did experience a frequent deep dull throb on the left side near all the scars from time to time, lasting a few minutes to a few hours. I did not know it at the time but this vague and widespread ache accompanied many of the changes, both good and bad, that were going on within the thin and fibrous tunica albuginea. For this reason I continued to periodically experience this dull ache even while I was responding positively and successfully to my own therapy program. Later I came to realize that the ache meant something was happening within the tissue in and around the scar. After I started to notice a number of good things happening to me (softening of the scar, reduction of curvature, return of lost length), I realized that this peculiar dull ache meant that the internal tension of the soft tissue was changing in the right direction. Thus the dull ache I noticed was caused by changes in the internal tension of the tissues, and would be felt whenever there was a change in tension, either as a worsening or improvement of my PD.

Wait and See, or PD Russian Roulette

During this time I read over and over again in all of the standard medical texts that the most common procedure to treat the early case of PD is to simply observe the condition, and monitor it for progress or regression.

The idea is, about half of the cases of PD get better on their own; those who will experience spontaneous recovery will usually do so within the first or second year, and for these men any treatment is just a waste of time. The problem is, no one can predict who is in that lucky 50% group whose PD is just a brief and temporary scare. For the 50% of men in the unlucky group, their PD usually worsens and eventually stabilizes in wildly various degrees of penile deformity, impotency, and personal defeat. For these men, surgery is performed when the symptoms get so bad that doctor and patient think the risk of surgery is better than enduring the hellish life into which a man is placed by his PD.

This "wait and see" phase of medical treatment seemed like a bad idea the first time I learned of it. I thought immediately that no one could benefit from this therapy concept except the surgeon who was simply waiting for men's PD scar to "ripen" sufficiently. Intuitively, I just could not accept the idea of doing nothing for my problem, although that seemed to be the only option available.

There were few to no counter-forces or opposing opinions concerning PD presented in the standard medical literature. Standard medical thinking has a closed attitude toward Alternative Medicine treatment of PD, and this pushed me forward when there was really no good reason to do so. All information pointed in the same therapy direction and to the same sad and limited conclusions:

1. Non-treatment; wait-and-see for first 12-24 months after onset.

2. Use of a short list of drugs that have only lukewarm enthusiasm and spotty acceptance within the medical community.

3. Brief, minimal vitamin E usage at the onset of the problem. No differentiation is made between synthetic and organic forms of vitamin E.

4. Surgery, the ultimate and only "sure cure," although even surgery has frequent (40-50%) and considerably severe drawbacks and side-effects of impotency and/or worsening of the original deformity of the penis.

While these choices were not very encouraging or uplifting, what made them even less desirable was that none of these options seemed to be supported by good end results. All information indicated that if you faithfully did what your medical doctor told you to do, you were still in a lot of trouble, except if you were in that lucky 50% group.

Anger and Frustration amongst the Men

I did not know it at the time, but I was becoming infected with the same attitude of defeat and hopelessness that is so common among men with PD. If you do not believe a very real gloom and doom attitude of defeat limits the thinking of the PD population, just visit an Internet PD discussion forum or chat room. There you will find men who are despondent about their problem, confused about many facts concerning their anatomy and their condition, yet almost eager to authoritatively inform anyone who asks for information that there is no successful medical PD treatment.

If you want to witness a real outpouring of anger and irritation with life, go to a PD chat room and inform the other members that your PD has improved with an Alternative Medicine procedure. You will be descended upon by a small and faithful group of men who will attack you personally, and refute your claim for success. Their position of denial is taken simply on the basis that this is what they were told by their medical doctor and what they have read from medical sources. You will be called a liar, a cheat, a fool. The favorite attack is to assume that anyone with a positive thing to say is attempting to sell something to the group, and is therefore a "shill." If you attempt to explain yourself, you will be given little opportunity to actually discuss your ideas or experiences. The attack will be directed to your intelligence and morality, not to what you have done.

My PD started while I was practicing acupuncture in an Alternative Medicine clinic with several like-minded holistic MDs. After informing them of my problem I assumed they would easily develop a good list of therapies to use. To my surprise none could offer any alternative treatment suggestion beyond simply expanding on the usual vitamin E therapy. I found this interesting and very discouraging. Here were three medical doctors who devoted a large segment of their careers to successfully treating a wide variety of health problems, from allergies to herpes zoster, with a wide array of simple to exotic naturally occurring therapies, and we all were stumped by PD – initially.

My Florence Nightingale

It was actually my wife, a nurse, who began the process of investigating alternative PD therapies on the Internet. She read into the early hours of the morning, reviewing studies and papers, making copies and handwritten notes about anything she could find about PD. She quickly found there were many more encouraging ideas and information coming from the area of Alternative Medicine than from traditional medicine. In the morning she would stack a pile of computer printouts on the kitchen table for my review and education. I, however, was already infected with the common PD viruses of defeat and hopelessness. She tried to show me there were a lot of good possibilities to treat my PD, but I did not have much early interest in what she was discovering. Over a period of time I was overwhelmed by her dedication and interest in helping me – far greater than I was interested in helping myself. After finding perhaps the tenth pile of notes one morning, it finally occurred to me that I should do all I could to get better for her sake, as well as my own. I will be forever grateful for her love and for her confidence in my recovery.

After plunging into the deeper levels of research information from around the world, I saw a pattern that gave me an idea to explain why there was such wide variability – even contradiction – reported when PD research was being done with Alternative Medicine products. Most often, when reading about a research study of vitamin E, acetyl-L-carnitine, MSM or similar therapies, I noted three basic differences between the ways these products were being used. In the research world of the medical doctor and in the non-research world of Alternative Medicine, these products were used in an entirely different way. These differences could easily account for the difference in clinical results both report.

1. Synthetic or altered products were being used in medical research. Alternative Medicine is almost always practiced using naturally occurring products, along with all the naturally occurring vitamins, minerals, and enzymes that would typically be found in food.

2. Low doses of vitamins were used in research that simply followed the Recommended Daily Allowance (RDA) for it, compared to the much higher therapeutic doses usually used in Alternative Medicine.

3. Only one single product was used in a research project, naturally. It would be bad research if other products were being used at the same time, since it would not be possible to identify which of the several products were responsible for any improvement. In the non-research environment of an Alternative Medicine office it is done differently. Results are important. In Alternative Medicine practice it is common to use several different therapies to simultaneously treat the problem from different directions. Very little, if any, thought or concern is given to determining which of the several different therapies were "working" on the problem, and which are "not working." Only patient progress matters in the real world, and so that is the guiding force in determining how to proceed with patient care.

These are huge differences between the research environment of testing ideas and possibilities, and the clinical environment of treating real patients. Taken together, these three factors can explain the significant variations in Alternative Medicine results as are usually reported.

The average medical researcher might not appreciate the importance of these differences between testing individual Alternative Medicine therapies and the actual use of these same therapeutic substances in the real world. And this difference just might explain why the results between of the two approaches are so often variable and contradictory.

Research vs the Real World

The value of good research cannot be overstated, yet it is not of much immediate concern to the man with PD. While the arguments blaze in the research field about surveys and studies, the man with PD watches on the sidelines while his life, family, and sense of dignity erode. It is difficult to be patient or understanding about the complexity of clinical research when your marriage is falling apart because you cannot perform sexually. What works will always win out over theory. A man with a sick penis has a very narrow focus of interests.

It was my opinion then, and still is now, that it is not important which of several individual PD therapies is primarily supporting the tissue repair process, so long as progress is being made. A man with PD does not want to be a guinea pig in a research project. He wants to get well. He wants to feel like a man again, and he wants to forget he ever heard of PD.

With these realizations I gained hope that perhaps there was something I could do to help myself.

Getting Started with Care

After making the easy decision to start my Alternative Medicine therapy plan with vitamin E, the difficulty was in determining which to use from the hundreds of available vitamin E brands. More time researching the different products pared the list down. Phone calls followed to representatives at home offices of those same vitamin manufacturers, then review, reading and comparison of loads of data. These further investigations lead to a small list of rather exclusive "boutique" companies that specialize only in this one single vitamin. After interviewing the company presidents and their key people, I finally felt good about going with a very small company from Tennessee that is headed by Andreas Pappas, MD, PhD, who does clinical research at the University of Tennessee; he is considered by many to be the world's leading authority on the subject of vitamin E. The other company that came in a close second has a strong and well-deserved reputation, the world famous vitamin E pioneer manufacturer and maker of Unique E, the A. C. Grace Company. I started to use both of these on alternate days, just to make sure I was getting all of the best I could find.

This type of time consuming and exhaustive investigation was done for each of the various "discoveries" I made for Peyronie's disease treatment from the universe of Alternative Medicine. I worked my way steadily through piles of information and data that applied to various aspects of PD. I was on a mission, and the work was easy because my PD was getting worse.

Slowly and deliberately, over a period of slightly more than a year, I found many nutritional and Alternative Medicine products that scientific literature indicated had limited and variable therapeutic merit, and also located what I felt to be the very best companies that offered these supplies. None of these individual therapies represented the absolute answer to treating PD, but then again, nothing is ever a sure cure for this problem. All I was looking for were those Alternative Medicine therapies that had undergone adequate scientific scrutiny and demonstrated sufficiently favorable and positive findings in at least half of the trials they were subjected to – even when the other half indicated that they were ineffective – because all medications and techniques studied so far also show the same confusing contradictions of findings.

Those natural and complementary therapies that demonstrated promise less than half of the time were not taken seriously and were never tried in my personal initial treatment plan. At this point in my care I did not feel like being a PD guinea pig. I knew that time was an important issue for me, since the longer any health problem continues the more difficult it becomes to treat. I just did not want to waste any time with worthless and totally unproven and untried therapies. What I was looking for, and finding, was a solid list of Alternative Medicine therapies that at least worked more than half of the time in scientific studies. This became the foundation upon which my therapy plan was based.

It seems to be the nature of PD that if you learn of a treatment or product that produces good results to correct the problem, you will find an equal number of reviews and tests that say the opposite. This is the way of life with PD, and the basis of the frustration and difficulty in dealing with this problem. Using my simple "50% or more" screening method, I found a fair number of therapies to work with, all of which have shown promise in several studies and failure in others.

Part of my reason for not being too concerned with those therapeutic failures is in knowing that many times research is done with nutritional products that are synthetic, or simply used improperly or ineffectively during the testing process. So many times a study will show that a rather well researched product that has earned high marks in the Alternative Medicine community will fail to demonstrate the same results during laboratory tests. The reason for the failures is later found to be due to simple issues (use of synthetic nutritional products, lower dosages than are usually used, or isolation of only one element of a nutritional therapy without use of its typically occurring synergistic counterpart) that would not usually occur if the research was being conducted by someone more comfortable with Alternative Medicine concepts. I proceeded with my own treatment assuming those research results that showed positive findings were probably conducted with better products and more aggressive controls than were the studies that had negative findings.

Choosing the Best Companies and Their Products

As I investigated the therapies with the greatest research promise and worked with the best companies that produced those same therapies, I slowly added to my therapy plan. I started with the best vitamin E I could find, and then I quickly added the best vitamin C because anyone who uses Alternative Medicine knows that these two work hand-in-hand enhancing each other's function in the body. From there I added a great MSM product because of what I knew about the function of sulfur in soft tissue repair and healthy scar formation. Those were the easy therapies to begin care. After that point I had to dig to find the right direction to take. Early in care with just three therapies at work, I noticed no significant changes in my PD, and perhaps some worsening.

Further investigation led me to include PABA, a naturally occurring member of the B vitamin family, and the foundation for the drug POTABA. You see, POTABA (the drug) is just a modification of PABA (the vitamin). What actually was demonstrated in research testing of POTABA is that it has been shown to be effective in a fairly good percent of cases, but caused significant digestive complaints. And of course, since the drug, which is much more profitable to sell, did not do well in medical testing, no interest is shown to working with PABA, which would not be as profitable to sell. For all these reasons I added the best PABA I could find to my therapy plan, and still kept on taking the vitamins E and C and MSM, as well.

Over a period of a few months I also added some Japanese campo herbs and bromelain to my treatment plan, and later quercetin was included. I used a very simple and direct non-needle acupuncture treatment, also. It was at about this time that I detected a noticeable and welcome change in the size and density of my PD scars. At first the changes were temporary and minor, lasting only for a day or two, followed by the scars returning to their usual size and hardness.

Although the improvement fluctuated, my enthusiasm and confidence did not. This was the first time I noticed any positive change in the scars, allowing me to conclude the plan was finally large enough to generate a synergistic effect that was headed in the correct direction.

During the second half of this first year of discovery and investigation I added nattokinase and serrapeptase, both well-researched and proven protein digesting enzymes that have been used for centuries in the Orient for a wide variety of fibrotic problems. The idea behind selecting the protein digesting enzymes was that the PD scar is composed of a defective network of fibrous protein-based material; the protein digesting enzymes should work to remove any abnormal tissue from the body. DMSO was next added to my plan of attack, along with topical vitamin E and a unique copper peptide product from the cosmetic's industry well-known for its ability to reduce superficial scar tissue and improve the health of soft tissue in general.

Lastly, as I was nearly cured and well on my way to normalcy, I put together a truly wonderful and multi-level dietary approach for the treatment of PD. The details are found in Chapter 5, "Diet and PD."

With each later addition to my therapy plan I noticed additional changes in the physical nature of my scar, along with reduced curvature and regaining of lost dimension. My confidence and enthusiasm continued to grow as one by one my scars began to disappear. As I put together the last of my therapy program it became more and more difficult to determine if the newer therapies were actually contributing to positive changes since there was less and less a problem to use as a measure of success.

Healthier in Many Small Ways

There seems to be another benefit to the therapy program I follow, that was totally unintended but no less appreciated. After a few months of faithfully following an aggressive plan of nutrition, energy enhancing exercises and acupressure therapy, people noted other changes in me. In time I also recognized both large and small unrelated benefits to my overall health.

During all of the 59 years of life my fingernails were weak, brittle, and heavily ridged. Now that has all changed; they are stronger, thicker, the ridges are gone, and even the nail bed has more rounded contour. My hair is less gray than before and it is thicker; my barber notes that I have developed a cowlick toward the back of my head that I used to have when I was a kid, 45 years ago. My hands and feet are no longer cold as they once were, and last winter my wife reminded me that I did not complain of the intense pain I usually had if I went out in the cold without wearing gloves. My digestion has improved, with less bloating and abdominal pain and less gas. I have better stamina and do not tire as easily when doing yard work.

These unintended changes and benefits indicate the PD therapy program I follow is working to help me become healthier, with my body responding positively in many different ways. I really don't care that I have darker hair on my head. But it is really exciting to know my body is functioning better – especially in regard to sexual function – and a case can be made that my immune system and capacity for cellular repair are able to do things for me now that were not being done before. As a result I think it is possible to live a longer and healthier life because of what I am doing for my PD.

After more than a year of faithfully following an aggressive therapy plan, my PD completely healed. This is based on the total absence of scar tissue, no pain at any time, no loss of sexual function, return of lost dimension, and no curvature during erection for more than a year. I hesitate to declare a complete cure because PD can and does recur. Nonetheless, I have decided I will continue to follow this same basic therapy program forever, just because I feel better being on my program of care.

Not a Guide, Just an Example

With this overview of my experience with PD, and successfully treating it with Alternative Medicine methods, the reader should have a better idea of what one person's experience has been. This information is not intended to serve as an outline or format of what will happen with anyone else. The story and experience of any man with PD should only be used to educate and illustrate what can and does happen, but not what will happen to anyone else. Other men's experiences with their PD only illustrate that PD is a hugely variable problem in which anything can and often does happen. Do not make the mistake of using someone else's experience to measure and compare your own. Doing so will likely disappoint and frustrate you. You and your PD will follow a unique path. How do I know this? Because, in talking to hundreds of men about their situation it soon became apparent the details of no two stories were alike. Everyone with PD has variations with (excuse the pun) twists and turns, which are unlike anyone else's experience.

Be prepared for a unique journey with your PD. Hopefully, using some of the information and ideas expressed in this book, your encounter with the terrible little scar that makes life so miserable and complex will be shorter and more tolerable.

Chapter 2 – Variability of PD Suggests Treatment Strategies

Ω - To live a better life, be happier and healthier in spite of your PD, and increase your chance of successfully treating it …

… you must understand the nature of the PD scar and why it changes. The very fact that it changes at all suggests "activity," "modification," "transformation," and "opportunity." Push this variable nature of the PD scar in the correct direction with the proper treatment strategy and you could have healing taking place. That is what this chapter begins to explain.

Let's place a little-mentioned issue about Peyronie's disease clearly in the open:

Most men notice their PD scar changes back and forth in some way over time – occasionally just a little, and other times a lot – perhaps for the duration of the condition. These changes occur not only during the initial phase of PD, when the scar first develops and changes the most and fastest. These changes are also observed in well developed and mature PD scars.

A PD scar can periodically alternate between different physical states and presentations like the tide, except the scar does not change with regularity or predictability. Back and forth it ebbs between smaller and larger, or softer and harder, or flatter and rounder, or easy to find and difficult to find, or smooth edges and surface and rough edges and surface, and so on. The PD scar has a different tempo over time, one that usually cannot be anticipated by the non-observant person. But to the observant person, who has taken the time to learn how to monitor the physical characteristics of his problem, some predictability and order can be found in these physical scar changes.

Scar, Nodule, or Plaque – It Is All the Same Thing, But Changing

If you experience small or large and slow or rapid changes in your scar, you are not alone. That is the good news: you are not imagining things. But, even more good news: It is my opinion that this unpredictable variability is actually a positive quality of your scar. This chapter will explain why you should be pleased – even delighted – your PD scar changes every so often.

Almost every man I have communicated with about his PD, and there are perhaps over a thousand by now, have reported that his PD scar is not static. The vast majority admit the scar will unpredictability change size, shape, density or even the appearance of location from time to time. A few will claim their scar does not change at all. When questioned these men admit they do not pay much attention to their scar for the most part, and often make a comment like "I am not good at that kind of thing, you know, I don't have a good sense of touch." **PDI** estimates that around 80% of men we communicate with experience variability and unpredictability of the physical state of their scar.

This notion that the scar of PD is not static first seemed odd and rather impossible when I first started to make observations about my own situation.

Perhaps it strikes you that way, too. But please note that physical variability of the scar is consistent with the overall nature of the problem of PD. Along this line of thought, it would be more surprising if the PD scar did not, in fact, change. Most everything about PD is unpredictable, variable, and non-conforming, why not the physical condition of the actual scar?

Change is Good

To appreciate what the variability of the scar suggests about Peyronie's disease in the larger picture of treating PD, first consider a comparison which anyone who has raised children will relate. If you had a child who had perfect manners, pleasant and friendly attitude, with beautiful behavior one minute, and then he changed into an irritating, terrible, loud, and rude person the next minute, you would, of course have a real problem. Part of the difficulty would be in trying to understand why the child displayed such drastic and variable change. Your thinking might be something like this: "This child can and does show good manners, self-control, and pleasant adult-like behavior on some occasions. He is capable of good behavior, and so I will expect more of this good behavior, perhaps even all the time. All I have to do is figure out what causes the good behavior and promote that, and then figure out what causes the bad behavior and minimize that." And so it would also be reasonable to think the same about the PD scar.

Since the PD scar can and does change in many ways on its own, sometimes for better and sometimes for worse, just like a child, the challenge is similar. *Consider that perhaps, just perhaps, to treat a PD scar, the task is simply to determine how to influence the scar to promote the favorable phase of scar activity by minimizing and avoiding the circumstances that seem to promote the unfavorable phase of the scar cycle.*

One of the main topics of this book is about just this subject: How to influence this good/bad cycle of the PD scar.

The challenge then becomes to analyze what is going on in your life – what you do, what you don't do, what you eat, when you eat, how you eat, what happens to you and how your body responds – that just might influence and exert some level of control in the coming and going of the variable scar cycle. Once a person identifies the activities and things that influence the physical condition of the PD scar, it is a rather simple matter to continue to do those things that promote the favorable phase of the scar cycle and avoid those things that do not.

If the physical variability of the scar is a common finding in a high percent of men with PD, and you are not crazy for thinking that your scar actually is different from one time to the next, then why does the medical literature not report on this interesting capability of PD? If a PD scar can frequently change size, shape, density, definition (surface quality) in the penis – over a period of years, not just for a few days or weeks – then why didn't your family doctor talk to you about that? Why did you not read about it in the literature your urologist gave to you, or why did you not read about it on the hundreds of medical PD web sites you have visited during your own research? If you are not imagining things, why has someone not presented this information to you before now?

While researching the medical literature for current information about my own PD, and later while researching the literature to write this book, I could not find an authoritative source of information that mentions the tendency of the PD scar to change size, shape, density, and definition. No medical web site or report I have yet found discusses this common characteristic of the PD scar, as though the PD scar does not change. It is as if the medical research community is unaware of the many physical scar changes that most men with PD experience.

Information is Ignored

When I ask men if they have told their family doctor or urologist about the physical changes in the PD scar, I am often told they did mention the physical changes at least once, and usually a few times; men do tell their doctors about these physical scar changes. And when I ask about the doctor's response to this important information, I am consistently told something interesting. I am told the doctor does not say much about this bit of information. The doctor might ignore the information all together like it was never spoken, or sometimes I hear that the PD sufferer is told by the doctor that he is mistaken; that he does not have a good sense of touch, or that he is imagining that his scar changes as he has reported.

Never have I been told that the doctor will take the information seriously, discuss the possibility or ask further questions to learn more about his patient's observations. No, I am told that the information is dismissed and ignored for the most part. So much for an inquisitive and probing scientific mind working in the average physician.

How can this be? Isn't every good doctor a scientist deep in his or her heart? Isn't the scientific approach to life a genuine and tireless curiosity about the unknown?

Don't all good scientists have a healthy curiosity? You would think so. Yet, when the average doctor is confronted by the average man with PD something different happens. The PD patient is met with lack of curiosity about a new and interesting piece of information that would tease and tantalize a curious scientific mind.

It is easy to understand why the average layperson is fascinated to learn the PD scar changes size, shape, density and definition for many years. However, the real life experience of the average PD sufferer is that he only observes his doctor's lack of interest when he is told about the scar frequently changing its physical characteristics. This must surely bother and irritate every man whose well-being is not given the attention and interest that should be coming from the curious scientific mind of his doctor. But there is a reason for this response. It is neither a good reason nor the reason you would like to hear, but is the only one that makes sense.

Are you ready for the answer that explains why the average doctor does not want to hear that your PD scar can and does change? Well here it is. The medical profession simply does not want to consider or acknowledge the periodic variation of the PD scar because that little fact disturbs and contradicts all of their comfortable thinking about PD, so they ignore it. They simply can't handle the kind of information that does not fit into their current explanation of PD. It drives them crazy. The unpredictable physical state of the PD scar unsettles their tidy little way of approaching the whole problem of PD and how they treat it. And so, they conveniently pretend it does not exist.

As a profession they ignore this everyday fact of PD life because it does not fit their contention that the scar is permanent and must be removed at great physical and financial cost if a patient wants to be normal or hope to have sexual intercourse again. If that seems like a rather harsh statement, it is.

It seems that the medical profession is so frustrated and confused by the whole issue of PD – just as the men who have the problem – that they cannot handle this truth about the PD scar and just pretend that it doesn't happen. They have a reason to ignore this aspect of PD. If they would acknowledge the PD scar is not like a skin surface scar, then they would have to start treating it differently.

Right now the medical community is in a comfortable state with PD. So many easy office visits are made in which not much is done, except to monitor and evaluate the scar. The doctor does not spend much time with the PD patient in treatment or active consultation. I have had many men tell me their medical doctor has never once felt or examined their scar! Can you believe it? The doctor is merely waiting for the problem to sufficiently worsen – meaning the poor guy with PD is adequately miserable and disgusted with himself and his life, so that he does not mind that surgery might further disfigure him – providing clear and legal justification for surgery.

Changes, Changes and More Changes All Around Us

1. Does the pupil of your eye change in size? Sure it does. It changes in response to light, or the absence of light. In the dark, it opens larger to let more light into the retina. In bright light, it closes down to prevent too much light from entering. Did you know that it can also change in response to fear, or happiness or to certain drugs, or to certain foods? Even though you did not know about these things happening in your eye as they occur, they happen anyway.

2. Does the shape and size of your penis change? Sure it does. It changes in response to stimulation from physical and mental signals. Did you know that an unborn baby boy while still in the uterus will get erections? Did you know that you get several erections a night, not related to a full bladder and not related to a sexual urge? This type of erection just happens because the body uses the erection to bring more blood to the penis and keep that organ healthy. Did you know that many men who are sexually impotent will sometimes still get these erections in their sleep? Yes, and even though you do not know about these erections that happen at night, they happen anyway, tens of thousands of times in your life.

3. Do your arm muscles get larger and firmer when you use them more? Sure they do. If your life changes and you suddenly must work harder for a long time, each muscle group will get larger in response to the work load that is placed on it. Did you know that when your muscles get larger, it is not because you get more muscle fibers, but the individual muscle fibers that have always been there just get bigger? What about when you break a bone and you cannot move while you are in a cast? Do the muscles of that area get smaller? Sure. We have all noticed that an arm or leg quickly gets smaller after it has been in a cast. Yes, even though you did not know about what goes on inside the muscle when you work harder, or not work at all, the muscles change in response to their environment.

4. Do your hands get calloused when you work on a rough surface over a long time? Sure they do. Most men experience heavy callus formation over the entire hand (brick layer), or perhaps just in one or two places if the friction is very specific (violinist). Does a person have to think about developing calluses, or perhaps do something special to make them appear? Nope, the body automatically creates them in response to local stimulation to protect the skin.

5. If you get a tooth pulled, do the teeth in front of and behind that space begin to move and shift to fill in the open space? Sure they do. The body attempts to fill the vacancy and balance the biting surface for better efficiency. Does a person have to think about how much to move each tooth? Nope, the body once again makes physical changes automatically.

6. When you break a bone, do you know where the calcium specifically comes from? Well, with this question, you probably don't. Just think about this to really appreciate this clever engineering. To heal a broken bone anywhere in the body, the calcium that is used to repair the break comes from the ribs! It would be dangerous if the calcium was taken from the skull, pelvis, spine or the extremities, since any calcium loss would weaken these structures. But calcium coming from the ribs would only make them more springy and flexible, which is the way they are supposed to be anyway. A flexible rib is not a really bad thing. As soon as the break heals, the calcium levels of the ribs are restored. Very clever, this body.

7. Do you sometimes think about a really great meal, and find that you are making extra saliva? Sure, it happens. The body once again is doing things automatically in response to a very small stimulus – just a thought – not needing direction or approval directly from you. Once again you respond to a subtle stimulus or environmental factor.

8. Have you ever been pulled over by a police officer on the highway for speeding? I wasn't in the car with you, but I know what happened: Your heart started to beat a little faster, and you took in a deep breath as soon as you saw the flashing lights in the rearview mirror. Your nostrils flared a little, your pupils dilated, and you got that common fluttery feeling in the pit of your stomach. You were angry that you were going to have to spend a lot of money on a ticket, waste time while the ticket was being written, and you were upset that you did not see him sooner so you could have avoided the whole mess. How long did all of this take? Most of your response was immediate, and again, you did not have to think about it. It just happened as your body responded to another kind of stimulus.

So then, with all these examples and a thousand more that could be cited, we should not be surprised to find that **the body increases, decreases, hardens, softens, and modifies itself <u>in many different areas of the body</u> without asking permission, as it seeks to change, respond and adapt to thousands of things in our external and internal environment.**

Thousands of spontaneous changes take place every moment in your body, some small or large, some simple or complex, some short or long term, some unnoticeable or obvious. Thousands of these changes take place at any given moment, and we know of only a few of them.

This brief discussion is to underscore the idea that your body is changing to a huge range of factors and stimuli all the time, without your control, without your knowledge, and without your input – they are just going on. The best we can do is to attempt to understand or interpret what is happening in an effort to understand the wisdom of the body.

Basic but Important Ideas to Ponder

Let's explore some very basic ideas about the PD scar – nothing terribly technical or scientific – just broad and general ideas about the nature of this problem. To do so, please be prepared for some strange and simplistic thoughts that are posed to put a few things in the right perspective.

- The PD scar does not have the man; the man has the scar. The scar is in the environment of the man; the man is not wrapped around the scar. The scar did not really come out of nowhere, or because of bad luck. Something is wrong or went wrong with the man to cause it to start. Further, something continues to go wrong, preventing the scar from healing and going away on its own like any other disease state.

- The PD scar is a very lousy thing, and makes life miserable, but it is just an expression of some abnormal function of the man, much like an ulcer. The scar is not a parasite in or on the body – like a tick or a leech – that can be eliminated and all is well. This is why when the scar is surgically removed it so often recurs. It is said that if a man who has had his PD scar surgically removed lives long enough, it will come back every time to every man. This is because the basic thing wrong with the man is not addressed by the surgical removal – he still has the same basic problem or flaw that started it all.

- This PD scar is not like the scar on your knee or your abdomen; this scar is a different animal. It seems to have a life of its own, changing from time to time and in different ways at different times. Even the childhood scar on your hand or your knee will slowly change over time, because the body always attempts to heal and repair to the best of its ability. But the PD scar is much different in terms of degree and speed of potential change.

- Newton's 1st law concerns a principle of nature called inertia, explained as **"The tendency of an object at rest tends to stay at rest and an object in motion tends to stay in motion with the same speed and in the same direction, unless acted upon by an unbalanced force."** Thus, another way of saying it is that objects tend to keep on doing what they're doing. In fact, it is the natural tendency of objects to resist changes in their state of activity or inactivity. Another variation of this concept was first proposed by the late, great, 20th century philosopher, Flip Wilson, who said, "If you keep on doing what you've always done, you'll keep on getting what you always got."

Putting it Together

Fasten your seat belt. Let's put some of these ideas together and see where they lead.

1. The PD scar undergoes structural or physical changes in about 80% of cases. It can and does change size, shape, density, definition, and location, sometimes all five, over a long time during the duration of PD.

2. The medical profession does not admit these changes can happen, and they certainly do not attempt to explain how it is possible. They ignore this fact, and they continue to have nothing valuable to offer the PD patient.

3. Men with PD say their scar goes through stages where it will change over a period of time, stabilize for a while, and then change again in the same way or a different way.

4. Newton's 1st law states in the more complete explanation, "...an object in motion tends to stay in motion with the same speed and in the same direction **unless acted upon by an unbalanced force**." If we continue with Newton's logic, the scar should constantly change or not change at all.

5. If the man has the scar and the scar does not have the man, and if the scar is in the environment of the man and the man is not wrapped around the scar, then it would seem logical to look to the man for answers about the scar, and not so much look only to the scar.

6. If the scar changes, and it does, it would seem that it is being "acted upon by an unbalanced force" somewhere or somehow within the body of the man.

7. If the unbalanced force that changes the inertia of the scar is within the man, then perhaps a good place to start is by observing and monitoring the environment that the scar is in – the body of the man who has the scar.

8. If the scar is good one day (smaller, softer, less painful, creating less curvature), then the environment should be examined to determine how it might be influencing the scar in such a favorable way. It would appear logical to continue doing those things to the body's environment that causes this favorable change in the scar's behavior. These positive actions could serve as the basis for a successful treatment plan for PD.

9. If the scar is bad one day (larger, harder, more painful, easier to find, creating more curvature), then the environment should be examined to determine how it might be influencing the scar in such an unfavorable way. It would appear logical to modify or discontinue doing those things for and to the body's

20

environment that causes this undesirable change in the scar's behavior. These avoidance actions (what you should not do) could serve as the basis of a successful treatment plan for PD.

What Does this Mean to the Man with PD?

Based on all of the above, it should be apparent that it is considered a good thing your scar changes, and a really great thing if your scar changes a lot. You should be very pleased that your scar is capable of change.

Why? Because it would indicate that the metabolism of the scar tissue is not so static and dormant that it will not respond to the correct treatment. A changing scar is already demonstrating that it is capable of responding to the various environmental factors of your unique body chemistry and physiology. A freely changeable and variable scar means that it should be capable of change in the direction that you would like it to go – once you figure out how to do it.

PDI has long held to the beauty of two extremely simple and basic observations that seem to have eluded the entire medical profession. The logic for the first goes like this:

1. If this PD scar is actually not the same as a skin surface scar, and it has other characteristics that are not like a skin surface scar, then perhaps the rules that apply to a skin surface scar do not apply to the PD scar, and perhaps it should be treated differently than a skin surface scar.

2. If the PD scar does change size, shape, density, definition and even location, then it is not at all like a static scar that occurs after an injury on the skin surface.

3. If the PD scar is different from a skin surface scar, then perhaps treating it like it was a skin surface scar is a mistake and this is part of the reason that the medical profession has not found a treatment for PD.

4. If the PD scar does change size, shape, density and even location, for reasons that are not understood at this time, then perhaps these changes can be directed and controlled if the stimulus for change were discovered.

Here is the logic for the second very fundamental observation about PD:

1. The PD scar does not have the man (the man is not attached to the scar), the man produces the PD scar due to some irregularity or abnormality of the man (the scar comes from the man).

2. The PD scar is not a foreign invader in the body (it is not like an insect that bites and attaches itself to the body). It is part of the man who made it out of or from his own body in response to an injury or stimulation to which he might be genetically prone. So in this sense the PD scar is an expression of the health and integrity of his body, much like an ulcer.

3. The presence of the PD scar indicates that something is wrong in the body who possesses the scar, since it is commonly seen as the overreaction of a natural reaction to injury.

4. Successful treatment should be directed to the man who has the scar, not the scar itself.

All of these ideas lead to a conclusion that greatly empowers a man with PD.

It might be truly possible to study his scar behavior, and determine if a relationship exists between his personal behavior and the broad environment of his scar. If, in the course of this study and investigation, he begins to notice a pattern of some regularity – even if it is not perfect – it provides a basis of anticipating responses of the scar behavior. It is then just a short leap to create a plan of action for treatment. This plan is simply a way to promote those things associated with reduced scar presence and avoid those things associated with increased scar presence. All of this leads in a direction that is favorable for controlling and perhaps even eliminating the PD scar.

The rest of this discussion concerns those things which might make it possible for you to control your PD scar.

Chapter 3 – What Causes the PD Scar to Change?

Ω **- To live a better life, be happier and healthier in spite of your PD, and increase your chance of successfully treating it ...**

... you must attempt to treat YOUR PD in the way that is right for YOU. Here is a discussion of the larger picture of those things that might be influencing the activity or metabolism of your PD scar, and therefore your life. This chapter discusses PDI's survey results that focus on those areas that appear to hold most promise for successful treatment.

If there was actually a really good response to the question, "What causes the PD scar to change?," the title of this book would be much different, and this particular chapter would be the largest instead of the smallest. The short answer to this question is that no one knows what causes the PD scar to change, but we are a lot closer to an answer than just two years ago.

It is the opinion of **PDI** that understanding the cause of the frequent changes in size, shape, density and definition (or surface quality) of the PD scar will directly lead to an improved treatment of this disabling disease. Since it is apparent medical research has not even acknowledged that the PD scar is capable of variable and ongoing periodic structural changes, no investigation has previously been done in this area by the medical community.

Once the existence of "the variable PD scar" phenomenon was first discovered by **PDI** in late 2004 we began studying it. We included several questions about scar variability in our online survey, and have been collecting data about scar changes from around the world ever since.

Now that a clearer picture of scar behavior is emerging from the survey data, another step can be taken to tentatively improve the treatment of PD. Our current theories and understanding are not complete, and certainly over time much more will be learned. However, we feel that we now know enough to ask better questions so that we can learn even more.

It would be wonderful, a dream come true, if this was the longest chapter of the book. Even though this is sadly the shortest chapter of this book, it is perhaps the most important.

Once you understand what is causing your particular PD scar to undergo its sporadic changes, you will suddenly be in control of the activity of "the enemy" and you will be able to guide him out of your life.

Collecting Data about Scar Changes to Help Us All

At the conclusion of this chapter I will ask you to do something that is very important. I trust that you will be motivated to spend just a few minutes of your time to join in this little project that might make a difference to the entire PD community – of which you and I are reluctant members.

A really great guy has been sending me a lot of questions lately about PD. Because he is very excited about his recent progress since starting his **PDI** program, he recently said in an email, *"I'm optimistic about the future and grateful for* **PDI** *which I view affectionately as a kind of secret concerned big brother collegial fraternity."*

With this "fraternity" in mind, held together by our similar burden in life, I ask that you take a moment of your time to consider the questions at the end of this chapter, and write an email to **PDI** giving us the benefit of your personal experiences and observations.

The information you contribute, when combined with information from many hundreds of others just like you, could easily make a huge difference in understanding this problem. After all, it is from the collective information developed through the **PDI** web site survey, and from talking to hundreds of men about what is going on with their individual problem, that the theories and ideas of this chapter and the rest of this book came into being. Help us and help yourself by sharing your ideas and hunches about PD.

Please, do it now before you make an excuse not to.

Preliminary Data Points in an Interesting Direction

From initial and ongoing **PDI** studies and surveys that started in the latter part of 2004, an interesting response pattern has emerged. Evidence is coming together that shows that change – both good and bad – of the PD scar might be a combination of different aspects of the daily diet.

The data that is being collected and reviewed points to a specific pattern of food choices that seem common among men with PD, which appears to keep the PD scar situation under a reasonable level of control. This pattern is best explained as a rather specific avoidance strategy. Apparently, the pattern of food elimination is simply a way of not stressing the scar or plaque with these certain foods, in a way yet to be determined. When the body is not stressed by these foods, the scar presence becomes minimized, occasionally so minimized as to disappear. The degree of actual reduction depends on many factors, some that we currently recognize and those that we do not. A very important factor that can be controlled and easily implemented is the combined use of enzymes and nutritional supplements as outlined in the **PDI** therapy strategy, as given on our web site.

First, Let's Consider Genetic Predisposition

Certain people are predisposed for one reason or another to certain diseases, for reasons that are beyond the scope of this book. For our purpose it is sufficient to note that some people have such a predisposition to diabetes. It is true that most everyone could become diabetic if they abused refined high carbohydrate food (sugar) long enough. Almost like working to become diabetic, prolonged abuse of refined sugars and high carbohydrate foods could result in anyone developing a diabetic condition sooner or later. However, some people do not need to abuse and overuse those high carbohydrate foods – they develop diabetes easily and early in life without much provocation. For these people, developing diabetes is an easy and fast process. And, there are those who are big sweet-eaters all of their lives who never develop diabetes. In either extreme, the ease of this process is based on the idea that some people are more genetically predisposed to diabetes than others. They develop the problem faster and to a greater degree than those who are not genetically predisposed. Thus, for them it is prudent not to eat too many high carbohydrate and refined sugar-based foods or diabetes might occur. Better safe than sorry.

Gout, a problem of protein metabolism that leads to a nasty type of arthritis, is another disease with a similar genetic predisposition. If a person has little or no gout predisposition, a great amount of rich and high-protein foods can be eaten with little or no problem. However, if a person is genetically predisposed, a relatively small amount of high protein foods will cause a terrible display of gouty arthritis, generally in the foot and the great toe specifically. You will notice in gouty arthritis that not only is there a factor of genetic predisposition, but a "target tissue" is also involved, just like with PD.

Get Ready, Here Comes the Good Stuff

Similarly, many forms of cancer, Parkinson's disease, balding hair patterns, and hundreds of other small and large health problems have been found to have underlying genetic predispositions. These genetic weaknesses can be triggered or aggravated by many **environmental** and **dietary** factors. **Similarly, it appears there could also be a dietary link in developing and/or interference of the self-repair of PD.**

- Does that sound absolutely crazy to you?
- Does all of this sound like the nonsense that your trusted MD warned you about?
- Does this fulfill the prophesy of all the guys on the PD discussion forums who warn that only kooks and crooks say PD can be helped, that you should just get used to looking like a "freak?"
- Are you now highly suspicious and uneasy with what you are reading?

Good. It means you are paying attention; I was afraid you were falling asleep.

Have you not read in respected scientific reports, from the AMA, from university hospital research facilities, from Mayo Clinic, from trusted government agencies, that certain foods should be avoided and others included in your diet in treatment of many diseases?

Long lists of foods and vitamins, developed by respected medical sources, are available to reduce the risk of this or that kind of illness: cancer, arthritis, diabetes, senility, Parkinson's disease, macular degeneration, all types of serious cardiovascular disease, and many chronic degenerative diseases. Sure, we know the news reports are full of this kind of information. After a while we block it out because it can be contradictory and confusing. But it is there nonetheless, and it suggests something to you about the dietary treatment of PD.

All over the news it is reported daily that diet not only affects heath, but certain specific dietary groups (fats, grains) are vital to health and wellness. Even certain specific foods (broccoli, sardines, or the burnt fat on a charcoal grilled steak – how's that for specific!) are found to be good and/or bad for certain nasty diseases.

So just stop here for a moment. Think about these little connected thoughts. Try to approach this idea without the prejudice of standard medical thinking. Approach it with an open mind, based on what you know for a fact from what is going on around you during your day.

What is being proposed is not exotic or complicated. It is profoundly simple, yet revolutionary because it has never been connected together in one place for your consideration, until now.

With a few minutes of truly independent thought it will make perfectly clear, simple, easy to understand, and logical sense to you: It is possible that diet can influence PD, maybe even your PD.

So, exactly, why is it so shocking or revolutionary that diet might affect the bump on your penis? Why? Because the noble medical profession has never said it, and all of the efforts of medical research are being spent looking for magic high cost drugs or additional high cost surgery to treat you with. They are too busy looking for exotic and expensive treatments which <u>they</u> can control. They do not want to look for simple and inexpensive things of which <u>you</u> can be in control. How about that for an answer, my friend?

Diet and Disease in General

If you are still skeptical about the possibility of using dietary measures as part of your PD treatment plan, please consider these common health problems.

None of this is complicated or difficult. In fact, these suggestions are so common place – from your medical doctor or your grandmother – that you do not even question this information when you hear it. So, why not PD, also?

Perhaps you know of someone who, or you yourself, has been advised by his medical doctor to make these simple dietary changes in these situations:

- **Anemia** – eat more red meat

- **High blood pressure** – avoid salt, eat more fish

- **Sore throat** – gargle with lemon juice and honey

- **Gall stones** – use an olive oil and lemon juice flush

- **Macular degeneration** – eat more tomatoes and carrots

- **Cold and flu** – eat oranges, garlic, take zinc

- **Bladder infection** – drink cranberry juice

- **Insomnia** – drink warm milk or chamomile tea before bedtime

- **Ulcer** – avoid vinegar and spices

- **Constipation** – use high roughage foods for bulk, drink more water

- **Cancer** – eat dark green leafy vegetables, reduce refined, preserved and processed foods, limit meat

- **Osteoporosis and broken bones** – drink milk and eat cheese

- **Complexion problems** – avoid refined and processed foods, sugar, greasy foods

There are, of course, many more common examples of how diet and food are used without any hesitation or doubt in other similar situations. Medical practice used to consist primarily of dispensing this kind of knowledge as a fundamental way to treat most every disease.

By now you should be most enthusiastic and excited at the mere possibility that you can help yourself rather than pine away about how lousy your life has become since PD visited you.

I sincerely trust this little review of common medical information has lit a fire under you. Armed with this insight, it should be easier to take charge of your problem and have confidence in your ability to do something about this terrible problem. Once you become active and involved in your recovery, you will feel more empowered and enthused than at any time since you first heard the ugly words "Peyronie's disease."

Genetic Predisposition to PD

Some men appear to be so genetically predisposed to PD that little or no physical injury or provocation is needed to start the problem; they develop PD without any apparent injury. Some not only develop PD, they develop similar fibrous tissue infiltration and fibrous tissue densities in other body parts like the hands and feet, all with names as similarly exotic as Peyronie's own disease.

What this discussion proposes for your review is that perhaps all of us with PD have abused – some of us more than others – certain dietary "laws" or factors without being aware that they exist for us. Let us suppose that a subtle dietary abuse added sufficient metabolic stress to your body. As a result the tissue of the body, in the penis, reacted with a full-blown PD response that occurred without much physical injury or outside help. With this added metabolic or dietary burden the PD then developed rather easily. It just snuck up on us one day after a little unimportant bump that went unnoticed.

Diet Caught by Surprise

We did not start out looking for a dietary connection to PD. It just appeared on its own and has not gone away. A dietary influence seems to be present in most PD survey results we see, suggesting some level of possible influence.

It is hoped the case has been made that diet and PD might be associated. If so, we are pleased. The next chapter will go into considerable detail explaining how to make several small and simple changes in your diet to determine if your PD scar could respond in a favorable way. If that turns out to be so, when coupled with the vitamin and enzyme changes that are also suggested by **PDI**, additional scar changes might also develop for you – sometimes even in a major way.

Questions about What You Eat and How You Eat

This is a different kind of information request than what you will find in the survey under the "Self-examination" and "**PDI** survey" tabs on the **PDI** web site.

What comes next is a short list of areas of interest to **PDI** at this time. We ask that you write an email to **PDI** using www.info@peyronies-disease-help.com as an email address. Please keep your answers to the point and as detailed as possible with facts and specific information related to your situation. None of your answers will be published in any direct manner, only generalizations and composite data will be published later. Never will a name be given to anyone at any time for any reason. We maintain your total privacy and confidentiality as dearly as we hold our own. You are guaranteed it is a trust that will never be broken.

Provide just a few sentences to explain each question, please. If you think that you are about average for a particular question, then just give the number and say, "Average" or "Nothing special." If you find a special question you would like to expand upon because it is really important to you, or it applies to you in a major way, please give as many details as you can.

Here, for any and all to respond, is what we want to know about the way you eat and what you eat:

Question 1. Are you a fast eater or a slow eater? Do you chew your food well, or do you gulp it down without much chewing? *Normal*

Question 2. Do you load up your drinks of water and soda pop with a lot of ice? *— Yes* Do you prefer to drink cold drinks more than hot drinks? Or is it the other way around for you? Do you dislike cold drinks and prefer warm/hot drinks? *Cold/Yes* *√(c)*

Question 3. Do you avoid dairy products for one reason or another? Do you have an allergy or sensitivity to dairy products? Do you eat a lot of dairy *No* products? By that we mean, do you eat a small amount of many different dairy products, or a large amount of just a few dairy products (lots of ice cream but not many other dairy products, or lots of cheese but not many other dairy products)? *No*

Question 4. Do you avoid wheat products for one reason or another? Do you have an allergy or sensitivity to wheat products? Do you eat many bread and pasta products? By that we mean, do you eat a small amount of many *Y* different wheat products, or a large amount of just a few wheat products (lots of pasta but not many other wheat products, or lots of bread and pastry but not many other wheat products)? *No*

Question 5. Do you avoid sweet and sugary foods for one reason or another? *No* Or do you eat many different sweets and sugary food products? By that we mean, do you eat a small amount of a lot of different sweet and sugary products, or a large amount of just a few sugary and sweet products (lots of chocolate bars but not many other sweet products, or lots of Pepsi Cola or Coca Cola but not many other sugary products)? *Yes* *Medium*

Question 6. Do you eat a lot of raw fruits and vegetables? For the last several years there has been a lot of interest in improving health by eating better. As a result, many more people are eating more raw fruits and vegetables in salads. Is that true for you? How many salads do you eat a week? The same goes for raw fruit, like bananas or grapes or whatever. Do you eat more raw fruit than you used to or more than you see the average person around you eating?

Question 7. Do you have any unusual dietary habit or way of eating that you know is different from most people? We want to know if you eat differently in some small or large way, so think about this for a while. What are listed next are just a few examples, so use these just to get your thinking going in the right direction. Do you do anything like this: *Yes*

- Put black pepper on a lot of foods you eat, even food other people never put black pepper on? Use loads of black pepper?

- Use a lot of ketchup? Do you use more ketchup than the average person? *Yes*

- Do you drink loads of water or any other drink with your meal? As examples: several cups of coffee, loads of soda with your food, several glasses of water at each mal when you eat? It doesn't make any difference what the drink is, just that you drink a lot when you eat. *Yes*

- Loads of butter on your food? *not*

- Really eat a lot of greasy foods? Loads of French fires, batter fried foods, grilled meats that are greasy? Do you prefer fried foods? *no*

- Eat a lot of high fat foods in a day? Are you a big cheese, meat, butter, and fried food eater? *No*

- Hate vegetables so much that you hardly ever eat anything green? *No* Only things you eat are meat and potatoes, both fried if possible?

- <u>Anything about what and how you eat that you know makes your diet different from the average person</u>?

Send an email with your answers to these six questions to:
www.info@peyronies-disease-help.com

30

Chapter 4 – Evaluate Your PD Scar Like a Scientist

Ω - To live a better life, be happier and healthier in spite of your PD, and increase your chance of successfully treating it …

… you must not ignore the problem that is ruining your life, you must become the master of it. To begin that process it is essential to have a very good idea of the size, shape, density and definition of your scar. This does not happen through casual observation, but by approaching the scar as a scientist would.

Whoever said "Ignorance is bliss" must have been happy because that is a very ignorant statement. Remaining ignorant in certain situations might be tolerable, but not when it comes to Peyronie's disease.

From the ongoing **PDI** survey analysis, it is apparent the current definition of PD might be in need of revision. Our study of PD suggests that information about scar variability is being ignored. It seems no one in the medical community has noticed this missing pieces in the PD puzzle, yet they attempt to put it together anyway. This ignored information has been most helpful in expanding our understanding of PD; this same information has been most helpful for the development of our new theories for care.

The intent of this chapter is two-fold: To expand your knowledge of the small but important details of your PD problem. Secondly, to guide the reader who wants to begin an Alternative Medicine PD therapy program to a logical starting point. With the data you will be shown how to collect, you will know far more about your particular problem than ever before.

To treat your PD scar and deformity successfully you must learn all that you can about its unique characteristics, <u>its behavior</u>, as well as the general state of health of that area of your body. By "behavior" is meant, what seems to make it physically different – it can shrink, soften, and become hard to locate, or the opposite, it can enlarge, harden, become sensitive, and very obvious. Thus, the more you understand about these aspects of your PD, the better position you will be in to control it.

This chapter will describe the process of collecting information about your scar and its behavior. If your conservative treatment makes progress, you don't want to come to a time when you ask yourself, "Is that scar getting smaller, is my penis less bent, or am I just imagining things?"

Collect and record the details of your PD problem at the beginning of care – and periodically afterward – so you will know exactly what is going on, or not going on. The data we ask you to collect is important for two primary reasons:

1. If you do not have a good PD therapy program and are not actually making progress, you might fool yourself into thinking that something good is happening, when it is not – and you needlessly continue with the wrong therapy plan.

2. If you are making progress with your therapy plan but it is very slight and slow, you might not notice small and subtle changes in your condition – and you might modify or quit a good plan even though your PD scar has improved.

A "Scar" Like No Other

As mentioned in Chapter 2, "Variability of PD Suggests Possible Treatment Strategies," the PD scar is capable of undergoing unpredictable degrees of physical change and modification from time to time.

Your project will be to collect detailed information about changes in the size, shape, density and definition of the scar mass. Also, as discussed at length in that same chapter, any of these changes of the PD scar strongly suggest encouraging possibilities about PD:

1. The non-static or variable condition of the scar demonstrates that it is not at all like a typical scar. Scar variation is good because it points to the potential to control and redirect that same change in a favorable direction, as well as minimize or prevent the unfavorable change. Thus by promoting the favorable changes and minimizing the unfavorable changes, PD scar changes might be influenced favorably – perhaps to the point of disappearance.

2. The body only undergoes change for a reason. It is reluctant to change without a reason to do so, as guided by the innate intelligence of the body as expressed in Newton's law. Therefore, we assume when the PD scar makes one of its frequent changes it is doing so in response to a situation or stimulus that occurs in the usual course of life. This assumption is based on the premise that the scar is not changing randomly or accidentally – it is adapting intelligently. This assumption suggests the high level of metabolic activity of the scar is dependant on, or triggered by, some internal or external factor that usually goes unrecognized.

These two possibilities highlight the need to be keenly aware of your eating habits, physical activity, behavior and emotion that influence the body. By knowing what is influencing the scar, the man is less the victim and more the master of the situation. Understanding scar behavior enables a person to manage scar behavior in a desirable direction.

Further, by applying this knowledge, it might be possible to limit the negative or undesirable phases of the scar. Desirable change, in the case of a PD scar, is intended to mean "gone."

Monitoring Your PD Scar

It is important to know what it means to monitor your PD scar. This idea does not suggest that you casually or idly make observations about the scar each time you urinate. This term also does not mean to check a single aspect of the scar, such as only the size or only the hardness of the scar. Lastly, it also does not mean to casually check the scar without preparation or thought.

Monitoring the PD scar means a complete study of all aspects of the scar is done each time you evaluate your condition, or that you perform no check at all. **PDI** finds that one aspect of the scar can worsen, while one or two other aspects improve. Thus, examine all aspects of the scar when you evaluate it. A complete check-up prevents you from being lead astray by partial data.

If only the one worsening aspect is evaluated, while ignoring the improved aspects, the wrong impression is created about the scar at that time. This then is ample reason to do a good job of evaluating the entire range of possibilities.

Working with the Collected Data

If you do not know where you are at the beginning of care, you will not be able to identify progress or lack of progress.

When the scar data is collected and compared over a period of time it can lead to better treatment decisions and appropriate modifications as changes warrant.

Using the most accurate and scientific information you can collect about your problem, your care will be guided intelligently and deliberately. Without this information you are only guessing.

Resistance to Dealing with Your Problem

When first presented with the actual details for the data to be collected, the most common response is something along the lines of, "Are you crazy or just weird? I can't be measuring, probing and tracing out pictures of my penis. The idea of taking a picture of my bent penis makes me feel like I am some kind of deviant. Is all of this really necessary?"

The short answer is, "Yes, it is necessary to do a good job. And, no, taking a picture of yourself is not deviant." Taking the picture is not deviant; it's what you do with the picture that determines if you are doing something that is not morally, legally or ethically correct. Since you approve of collecting this information or taking a picture in the first place and you maintain control over it, nothing inherently wrong should come of this information or photographs. If you do these things for your own good purpose and manage them appropriately, they are not "dirty."

Let's discuss some of the natural reluctance men usually feel when asked to do this kind of work with their genitals. And, interestingly enough, it begins with a discussion of women. To begin with, here's a real news flash: Women are different from men.

Yes, they sure are different, but not in the way you might have considered. Women seem to have a more realistic and mature attitude about the invasion of privacy to which they are often subjected. Though women are generally more reserved and modest than men, they learn early in life that private body parts are not really so private. Young girls discuss their private problems with family, friends and even strangers. They read about their private problems daily in all manners of public advertising. They shop for, work on, prepare for, mark calendars for, plan daily activities around, dress for, and deodorize, just because their private parts undergo a monthly menstrual function.

Women learn at an early age how to live their lives as though they do not even possess private parts, when in fact their private parts are exploding with activity several days every month. Young women learn their private body parts have not only the magical power of procreation, but that men go crazy for and fight for their private parts. Yet they must act like these private parts do not even exist. They accept the inconvenience and additional work that comes with being a woman. Sanitary pads and tampons, child birth, pelvic exams and PAP smears, lusting men, short skirts that ride too high, plunging necklines, breast feeding, and diaphragms all make their private areas a lot less private. Women learn to accept all of this, and more, as part of being a woman.

Some young women initially rebel against the changes that regularly and predictably take place in their lives. Within a relatively short time they submit when it is obvious little can be done to prevent what is happening to their bodies. Each eventually comes to a grumbling tolerance of these inconveniences as a part of their lives. They learn how to play the cards they have been dealt.

It's Just More Difficult for a Man

Men generally have no similar experience, training, or knowledge. They are totally inexperienced in thinking about or taking care of themselves and their genitals the way women must. Generally, men are totally unprepared to handle the stresses and demands of a problem in their private area. Men are spoiled in this way – this is good in general, but bad if you have PD. When something like PD happens to a man it is much more devastating to him than it would be if he had a woman's prior experiences.

Thus, when a man develops PD he comes just a little closer to knowing what it must feel like to be a woman, whose private parts are not so private. He is totally caught off guard and he suffers badly.

Does any of this make PD a less lousy problem to live with? No, not really. But recall how our female counterparts are able to deal with their own daily private part issues, and continue on like nothing is happening. This should put things in better perspective for those of us with PD. Like a woman who must make an emergency run to the store for yet another box of tampons, she takes it in stride. She accepts this as part of who she is and what her body has decided to do. She does not pout. <u>She deals with it and does not make a bad situation worse by fighting it</u>. Get the message?

Men with PD could learn a few lessons from women. If you don't believe me, just ask a woman.

Changes Reported in the PD Scar

Based on the most recent survey results conducted by the Peyronie's Disease Institute, the most common changes in the physical nature of their PD scar, reported by 154 men with PD, along with the percent occurrence of that change are:

1. **Size** (any dimension change in length, width or height of a scar) (81%) – from tiny bead size to 2-3 inch monsters.

2. **Definition** (ease of locating edges) (68%) – how easily the scar edge can be located; some are sharp and clearly defined, while others are broad, rounded-over and difficult to determine where the scar begins and ends.

3. **Shape** (64%) – a lot of scars seem lineal in shape, but round and irregular shapes are rather common.

4. **Surface quality** (perception of top surface of a scar, essentially a description of the smoothness or roughness of scar covering) (48%) – the fingertip is lightly glided over the scar to judge surface texture.

5. **Density** (degree of softness or hardness, or ability to detect "give" when scar is held between two fingertips and very light squeezing pressure is applied) (48%) – often a scar will seem to soften or get "mushy" as it is being absorbed or reduced during therapy.

6. **Location** (apparent scar placement change; most likely is actually multiple scars increasing and decreasing size and other qualities at the same time, creating this illusion) (43%) – approximate position seems to vary from time to time.

Of these changes surveyed, most men report that two or more different physical changes continue to occur. Only 28% of men note a single type of physical change in their scar has ever occurred.

Speed of Change

How rapidly any of these physical changes will occur varies considerably. The speed of change is variable from man to man, with some being "slow changers" and others "fast changers." In addition, the same man will report from time to time that he will experience phases in which his scar will change slowly and at other times the change will be much more rapid. The range of time in which physical changes have been reported is from hours to months, but is usually in terms of several days.

Frequency of Change

One of the hallmarks of Peyronie's disease is the extreme variability in all aspects, making it difficult to study, treat and live with. Mindful of this, the considerable variability of the PD scar should come as no surprise. Some men seem to be "infrequent" or "rare" changers, and others are "frequent" or "unstable" changers. As with the speed of change, many men report that their frequency of changes is also variable – sometimes more and sometimes less. The range of time in which physical changes have been reported is from days to months.

Written Records Are Valuable – Recollection Isn't Worth Much

It is common to hear men who are following a successful therapy plan admit to uncertainty about the degree of improvement at the beginning of care. They know the scar is smaller and harder to find, but do not have any real idea of the actual progress they have made. They also think the scar might be softer and feel different in ways they cannot explain, yet they have no way of comparing their current and past status.

Memories fail. Our recollection of things past is influenced by what we would like to be true; this is called selective memory, and we are all guilty of it. Hasty mental images and vague recollections are not good enough. The need for accurate information only becomes apparent after the fact, when it is too late to accurately recall. Please get used to documenting this most important work that you will soon be doing.

Anyone who has had children understands how memory fails with the passage of time. Your baby is young and does or says something that is so funny that you think you will never forget it. Yet, when the child is grown and long gone, you look through an old album or scrap book and find a picture or paper that jolts you because it presents proof of something you forgot. This happens to us all. You do not want to let that happen with your PD program because it can be a reason for failure – and no one wants to fail with PD.

Privacy for Your Data

Give some thought to where you will keep your data. Find a very secure and private place for the records and documents you will be putting together. If you are concerned someone might discover your sketches, pictures, tracings and measurements, find a very secure and private place for your deformities.

Equipment You Will Need

Just a few simple tools are necessary. You probably have most of it already, and what you do not have can be easily and inexpensively purchased.

1. Ruler

2. Tape measure

3. Pencil and paper

4. Digital or Polaroid camera to make 2-3 photos of your self

5. Calipers, or pliers or dull scissors to act as calipers

6. Forms to record data – provided at end of chapter

**You won't know for sure if your plan is working
unless you take the time NOW to evaluate
your scar and penile deformity before you begin therapy**

Important Suggestions for Monitoring Your PD Problem:

1. Write good notes. You might be starting a one or two-year effort, and small details can be forgotten or confused later.

2. Get help to determine the exact condition of the scar from your wife or significant other. Asking another person in your life for help in this area gives you the advantage of someone who can be more objective about your situation, to confirm or deny what you might think is going on. She will have an opportunity to discover something you might miss. Perhaps the most important aspect of asking for help is that you include your partner in learning about your problem in a unique way. This develops better understanding for what you are going through. Being more familiar with your problem avoids reluctance and hesitation to touch or hold your penis. This will go a long way

to avoid isolating yourselves from each other. With her being more confident and comfortable with you and your problem, she will be less fearful of hurting your penis and therefore more inclined to maintain sexual activity with you. Women have a strong sense of compassion and helping others. Her involvement appeals to her need to bond with you during this time. Lastly, you can take this opportunity as an exercise in being open, honest, and less embarrassed about your PD problem.

3. Be as accurate as possible with your data. Future comparisons must be meaningful to have total confidence in them.

4. Measurement and evaluation of the scar itself are best done while in the non-erect state. Usually very little, if any, of the scar can be felt when erect.

5. Use the centimeter scale if you are not good with measurements that involve fractions of an inch.

6. Use a caliper if you have one to measure your scar; a small plastic calipers is easily available from the Internet, sewing and fabric stores, and hardware stores, for $2.00-$4.00. Or you can use a homemade caliper. A simple substitute device that can be used in place of actual calipers is a pair of scissors, or something similar like pliers or tongs. **Carefully use the instrument** to measure the scar in two planes for an accurate determination of length and width. Feel the exact margins or edges of each scar. Accurately place one tip of the caliper on one side of the scar, and then the other tip on the exact opposite side of the scar. If you are using scissors, do not allow them move opened or closed while you get an accurate measurement of the distance between tips of the scissors with a ruler. Use the form at the end of this chapter to record your findings, and keep in a safe place.

7. Carefully trace the curve of your erect penis on a piece of paper. You will need this later for an accurate side-by-side comparison. Keep the pen or pencil perpendicular to the surface of the paper as you trace around the outer contour of the penis. Photos are not as useful as a life-size tracing.

8. Do not evaluate your scar too often. Once a week, or every other week, should be sufficient. Measuring too often should be avoided. If you are changing a certain aspect of your therapy (especially something in your diet) you might want to watch your scar more often for a while to observe how your body is responding. You can drive yourself crazy if you measure too often.

9. Understanding what is responsible for the changes your scar will make can be difficult. Always be aware of any change in your diet and environment.

It does take a while for the body to respond to dietary and environmental changes. You might possibly respond to something you did or ate in the last 12 hours or even the last two or three days. Time is required for changes to occur after a significant event, but how much time? Unfortunately this can be variable, and this is where the difficulty of interpretation of scar changes comes in. Accurate interpretation starts with good records.

10. Notice the suggestions or examples given below to describe the various qualities (softness, hardness, size, margins, etc.) of the scar. Each description uses the word "like" because they compare known standards which are as clear and precise as possible to you. Be creative and try to make it a personal thing that you can easily relate to later. These notes and comparisons are not going to be seen by anyone else, so be creative and as clear as you possibly can. They do not have to make sense to anyone but you; they must clearly document what you are feeling so that the next time you check yourself out you will have a meaningful gauge of progress. The trick is to ask yourself what the scar reminds you of, while you are actually feeling the scar.

11. It is difficult to have a sensitive touch while pressing down too heavily; a light touch often provides more information. Gently apply light pressure to the scar with the finger tips until you have an accurate impression or idea of the softness, hardness, overall density, or surface quality of each scar. Be as graphic or creative with your description as possible, so that each description will mean something to you many months later when you try to make a comparison.

Concerning Firmness of the Scar

If you only describe the degree of firmness as, "soft," "hard," "not hard," "softer than before," or "really soft" you will find later that these terms do not mean anything for comparison purposes. Even if you think you can use something like +1, +2, +3, and -1, -2, -3 to evaluate what you are feeling at each examination, you will soon find that these notations are meaningless. A few days after making this kind of determination you will find that you will question exactly what you meant by your "-2" entry.

You want to relate the exact quality of softness or hardness to something that you can compare later. You want to accurately measure progress, or lack of progress, against a reasonably established standard of softness or hardness that is reliable and measurable to you. Without this method of comparison you will be forced to try to remember the various qualities of softness and hardness that are long gone. This is called an "objective" standard. Size can be measured, a shape can be drawn, but how do you compare firmness?

Here are some examples to describe softness and hardness:

1. Soft like the tip my nose

2. Firm like the jaw muscles a few inches below my ear when I press my teeth together.

3. Gives to pressure like the lobe of my ear.

4. Firm like the boney end of the bent elbow.

5. Gives to pressure like a firm grape.

6. Mushy and really soft like an over-cooked lima bean.

7. Hard like a rock, does not give to pressure.

8. Gives just slightly like a bar of soft soap

9. Rubbery like "gummy-bear" candy

10. Gives under gentle pressure like a tennis ball

11. Gives under gentle pressure just like a marshmallow

12. As firm as the pad of muscle of my thumb when I make a fist

13. Density of an earthworm

14. Pretty firm like a carrot in my favorite stew

Concerning Edges or Margins of the Scar

Get an idea of the condition of the margins or edges of the scar(s). Are the edges really well defined and easy to locate; are the edges really blended into the surrounding tissue making the margins of the scar difficult to locate because they fade out? Be descriptive in how the edges or margins feel to you, just as you described the hardness or softness of the scar itself. The trick is to feel the edges or margins of the scar and ask yourself what it reminds you of.

Here are some examples to describe the scar margins and edges:

1. Sharp and well-defined like the front edge of my computer

2. Very rounded and broad like the front end of my computer

3. Fairly sharp edge, feels almost like it is a 90° edge

4. Almost sharp like the front opening of my CD player

5. Very rounded over like a bar or soap that has been used a lot

6. Difficult to locate because it seems to rise up gradually without a real beginning point like the back splash on the kitchen sink

7. Rounded edges like the buttons on the living room couch.

Concerning the Surface of the Scar

Get an idea of the surface, or definition, of the scar(s). When you run your finger over the surface, does it feel smooth and almost polished, or does it feel a little rough and irregular? Can you feel something like threads or fibers over the surface of the scar, like you were examining a coarse piece of cloth or the surface of a cantaloupe?

Again, try to imagine what this scar feels like and be as descriptive as possible, using imagery from your own experience.

Here are some examples to describe the scar surface:

1. Slippery and polished, like a greasy plate after dinner

2. Smooth like running my finger over glass

3. Almost smooth, feels just a little irregular like I am feeling a piece of wool

4. Slight irregularity, or fine bumpiness, like a terry cloth surface

5. Rather rough and irregular like I am feeling a piece of burlap

6. Irregular especially when I run my finger in a certain direction, then it feels almost "stringy" like the fibers of the scar are separated, but when I rub in the opposite direction I do not feel the separations and it feels pretty smooth

7. Almost smooth with irregularity like the surface of an avocado

8. Slick and very smooth like it is a piece of ice

9. Feels slightly bumpy like the cut end of a 2X4

Final Thoughts about Measuring Changes in Your Scar

When I was seeing frequent and dramatic, but fluctuating, changes in my own scars I tried to really picture what was happening under the surface of the skin. I got the very creative mental image that my largest and most damaging scar felt like a piece of ice that was melting in all directions at the same time. It felt like it was getting shorter, less wide and also flatter, just like an ice cube melting in the sun. However, this ice cube as I imagined it, was not made of regular ice. This ice cube was made of tightly wrapped strings or strands of twine – almost like a "string ice cube." As it melted and got smaller, the tightly wrapped strings got looser and looser, and it felt like there was more space between the strands. Also, as it got smaller the stringiness of the ice cube became sloppy and I could actually feel them move from side to side. The smaller it got the looser the threads became. Finally, that big scar just melted down to nothing. Eventually the scar had no height, width, or length, but for a few months, I could still feel the stringiness or looseness of the fibers where the lump used to be. In time, the fibers also went away. That was how I pictured it, in addition to getting good measurements of it.

Let your thinking and creativity go wild, because it will help your therapy.

On the next two pages are worksheets to copy for your data collection.

PLEASE NOTE, to protect your privacy when using this form:

1. There is no place for a name or identification.
2. There is no title or description of what this form is all about.
3. The term "SC" is used in place of "SCAR"
4. The term "PART" is used in place of "PENIS"

If your mother-in-law found this form, she would have absolutely no idea what it was about.

Sc 1, located_____

Date _____	Date _____	Date _____
Length _____	Length _____	Length _____
Width _____	Width _____	Width _____
Firmness _____	Firmness _____	Firmness _____
Margins _____	Margins _____	Margins _____
Change _____	Change _____	Change _____

Sc 2, located_____

Date _____	Date _____	Date _____
Length _____	Length _____	Length _____
Width _____	Width _____	Width _____
Firmness _____	Firmness _____	Firmness _____
Margins _____	Margins _____	Margins _____
Change _____	Change _____	Change _____

Sc 3, located_____

Date _____	Date _____	Date _____
Length _____	Length _____	Length _____
Width _____	Width _____	Width _____
Firmness _____	Firmness _____	Firmness _____
Margins _____	Margins _____	Margins _____
Change _____	Change _____	Change _____

Sc 4, located_____

Date _____	Date _____	Date _____
Length _____	Length _____	Length _____
Width _____	Width _____	Width _____
Firmness _____	Firmness _____	Firmness _____
Margins _____	Margins _____	Margins _____
Change _____	Change _____	Change _____

In addition to specific information, monitor and collect information about the overall condition of the part.

Use the following form to monitor the part

Date _____	Date _____	Date _____
Length _____	Length _____	Length _____
Circ'frn _____	Circ'frn _____	Circ'frn _____
Angle _____	Angle _____	Angle _____
Firmness _____	Firmness _____	Firmness _____
Locate sc _____	Locate sc _____	Locate sc _____

Date _____	Date _____	Date _____
Length _____	Length _____	Length _____
Circ'frn _____	Circ'frn _____	Circ'frn _____
Angle _____	Angle _____	Angle _____
Firmness _____	Firmness _____	Firmness _____
Locate sc _____	Locate sc _____	Locate sc _____

Date _____	Date _____	Date _____
Length _____	Length _____	Length _____
Circ'frn _____	Circ'frn _____	Circ'frn _____
Angle _____	Angle _____	Angle _____
Firmness _____	Firmness _____	Firmness _____
Locate sc _____	Locate sc _____	Locate sc _____

Date _____	Date _____	Date _____
Length _____	Length _____	Length _____
Circ'frn _____	Circ'frn _____	Circ'frn _____
Angle _____	Angle _____	Angle _____
Firmness _____	Firmness _____	Firmness _____
Locate sc _____	Locate sc _____	Locate sc _____

Chapter 5 – Diet and PD

Ω - **To live a better life, be happier and healthier in spite of your PD, and increase your chance of successfully treating it ...**

... you must learn if certain things you eat, or the way you eat, is somehow stressing your PD scar. If you follow the instructions in this chapter, you will soon learn if something needs to be changed in your diet – the food you eat, or the way that you eat. Not only might this improve your PD, it could also benefit your health and sense of wellbeing as well. This chapter will guide you in that process.

Ideas about PD and Diet Being Developed

This chapter is an introduction to **PDI**'s current ideas for influencing PD through diet; not the weight loss kind of diet, just a few simple modifications to your daily food intake to influence the scar. The intent of this chapter is to introduce you to a novel idea: What you eat and what you don't eat – simple food, common food – could actually influence the physical condition of the PD scar. If you are like the men who follow an aggressive Alternative Medicine therapy plan of vitamins, enzymes, and use different energy enhancement procedures as found on the **PDI** web site, and follow these dietary modifications, you might be in for a very nice surprise with your PD.

Basically, this dietary approach comes down to simply a list of foods to add and those to avoid in your daily diet, plus two simple modifications of how to eat. The avoid list is not that long, although it does cover some very popular foods. And most people find they already eat many foods on the "add" list. Therefore, most will have to make only a few adjustments to begin the program. If you find that you already eat and enjoy several foods on the "add" list, you are invited to eat even more of those. The more you follow the list the better. Usually 3-4 kinds of food are taken out of the daily diet, and a similar number added for just a few weeks. That's all. Nothing so crazy is asked of you that your world is turned upside down. Honest, this will not be painful, and it could change your PD and your life.

No absolute dietary rules can be stated with certainty that will improve your PD at this time. We will present to you the early guidelines that are based on information collected from just a few hundred men. We have coupled this information with the dietary traditions of cultures that are known for their robust health and good living well into old age. The results of this dietary concept looks promising at this time.

Please be curious enough about treating your PD via diet to leave your comfort zone for just a short while. Although the urges are usually strong to remain within the known and familiar, firmly resist the status quo of your eating habits. It will be necessary to harness your determination to beat PD, and direct that energy toward a few dietary changes that could influence your recovery from PD.

"...for just a few weeks."

A few paragraphs up the phrase "for just a few weeks" was used in describing how long you should sample this dietary modification. Did you notice that?

That phrase does not mean that this is the total length of time you might be eating this way. It refers to the length of time you should agree with yourself to investigate this dietary approach for PD, as a test to see how it works for you. At first you will be doing this merely as a test for a few weeks and then determine if it was successful. Usually three to four weeks is enough time for the tissue to begin responding to these chemical changes you are creating – if it is going to respond at all.

To follow this dietary program for only a few days or so, would be unfair to you and it is not fair to the idea being presented in this chapter. Doing less, cheating on the program, bending the rules, doing what is not allowed and in general being a wimp about disciplining yourself is an injustice to your goal of beating your PD.

We trust you are stronger and more mature than allowing a little food to beat you. No one likes to leave the dietary comfort zone they have established and followed for a lifetime. The thought of having a bent penis and no sex for the rest of your life should be a good motivator to try a few new things. Keep your thoughts and energy focused on your goal and do not allow any deviation from the simple eating plan you will find here.

Once you determine that, yes, eating this way does indeed help your PD, then you have a very nice problem: How long will you continue modifying your diet for the benefit of your PD? The answer, which is entirely yours to make, lies in one of three possibilities:

1. **Just stay with it.** Eat this way basically for the rest of your life, because your PD is improved or gone, and your general health is better since you started to eat this way.

2. **Experiment with the diet** after you are better. We suggest that you continue with your PD diet until you are sure that you are as good as you can be – you will never know until you try. Once you are as good as you can ever be, then you can experiment with it to see what you can get away with and not lose any of the penile improvement you made. Most men find they can deviate from the basic diet to a degree – once the total improvement has been made and they are feeling and looking great – and the PD will not recur. If it does recur to a small degree, then a few days or so back on a more strict form of the diet brings them right back to a straight penis and no scars. Each person seems to have a different tolerance level that must be explored. It takes some time to understand the interplay between your diet and your PD. Once you know what you can tolerate, it is easy. It is like someone with an ulcer: once the dietary rules are established by trial and error, it is known which rules can be broken, how much and how often. It becomes a simple matter of managing their dietary limitations. It is similar with PD.

We now have men who understand the connection between what they eat and how their PD responds. They no longer need to follow all the dietary restrictions they used to maintain their recovery. They know how to work their diet to keep ahead of their PD.

3. **Return to your old habits** in spite of success with your PD, because you find any dietary limitation uncomfortable and too difficult for you. And you can once again enjoy your favorite foods and your PD.

If this diet is not successful – and you really did a great job of following the program exactly as described for several weeks – you can at least feel satisfied that you tried to do something good for yourself. You will not hurt yourself by following any of the restrictions or additions. Most are common ideas about eating better, with just a slightly different combination of certain foods that make this different from anything you have seen.

Insanity and Your Comfort Zone

If you would find yourself walking in a northerly direction and getting colder all the time, but really wishing you were heading south so you could warm up, the logical decision would be to turn around. You would know that to change your situation you would have to take the action of turning yourself around. To continue walking north while wishing you were going south would be rather silly. This plays into the familiar definition of insanity as "Doing the same thing over and over and expecting a different result." If you want to explore changes in your PD, you will have to make some changes first.

We all have a rather large comfort zone taking in many aspects of life, and we usually protect it well. Even the idea of changing any part of your diet is uncomfortable. Great discomfort and resistance can be demonstrated over the small dietary changes needed to improve or resolve PD. It should really be as easy as determining which of these discomforts is more tolerable: temporarily leaving your food comfort zone or having PD. Most men decide nothing is as bad as having PD; a few dietary shifts are a small price to pay for a chance to return to penile normalcy.

Many people feel this way about putting out any effort for themselves: "Sure I want to get my life back to the way it used to be. I would do anything – so long as I do not have to inconvenience myself, or be uncomfortable and don't have to change anything that I enjoy doing." Not a good attitude, nor one inclined to be successful in the end.

All that is asked of you at this point is to find the determination to simply test these ideas to learn if you will respond in a favorable way; just try it for a while, and see what happens. That's not so threatening to the old comfort zone, is it?

47

Early Information about Diet and PD

Through collection and analysis of information from men from around the world we are beginning to see patterns and relationships that have never before appeared anywhere in the scientific literature. This is an exciting time for **PDI** and men with PD. While our understanding of the dietary connection is not complete, **PDI** is developing more interesting questions and ideas that are leading to even more interesting questions and answers. As this process develops and grows, the "PD dietary laws" should come into focus.

Most of the survey analyses point to a unique group of foods and ways that people eat that seems to influence the PD scar in some way that is positive or favorable – the scar simply gets smaller, softer and gets reabsorbed in a number of cases.

Aha! What does that mean, "...in a number of cases?" You mean your diet is not perfect and foolproof, not a 100% cure?

Nope, it is not, and probably can not be. Nothing in life is 100% perfect. We collected this data about the dietary association of PD while working under four primary handicaps:

1. **PDI** is working with total strangers from the Internet who only communicate sporadically by phone and email in an anonymous fashion, for the most part. They are in total control of their program from start to end, free to accept or reject the suggestions offered by **PDI**. We do our best to educate anyone who asks about our theories for improving the body's ability to heal. However, we have no way of knowing when, if, or how accurately anyone who comes to us for information is actually following our suggestions. In spite of these less than ideal circumstances, we get frequent reports of success in all areas of PD, from pain to bends to impotency.

2. Every man follows a slightly different course of care – his own. Each man comes to us with a variety of preconceived ideas and limitations that cause him to take a slightly different direction in his care; no two are alike. We exert no control in any way over the people with whom we work.

   The only similarity in the plans that are being used is that we ask each man to "Do as much as you possibly can, in as many different ways as possible, to gang up on this problem." In this way, we try to establish this one common denominator for each man to use the power of synergy to the best of his ability in his care. Because many men who use our ideas have limited finances, they use only a very limited number of supplements. They cannot afford to follow the more aggressive therapy plans that have a higher likelihood for success. Actually, only 5% or fewer of the men who employ our suggestions follow what **PDI** calls a "Large Plan," and perhaps 50% follow a "Medium Plan." On this basis, we often are working under less than ideal circumstances in which only modest synergy is created.

Others are men who are looking not only for miracles – they are looking for *easy* miracles to be thrown down on them. They quickly become discouraged after a few weeks of half-hearted effort, and quit. They tend not to blame themselves for their lack of success, but blame others.

3. We clearly admit at the start of this book, the start of this chapter, and everywhere else that is appropriate, that **PDI** is in the early stage of this work. Even though we are still refining our ideas, many men get good responses. We talk daily to men whose PD shows improvement after being non-responsive for years – until they began following the **PDI** therapy and diet suggestions.

4. We find that many who get good recovery fail to come back to tell us about it. It is human nature to get so busy with life that you do not follow up with what should be done. And so, our statistical collection is not as good as if done under a strict research setting. In spite of this, we note progress with these men who follow the **PDI** therapy concepts for the self-treatment of PD, as best they can do.

Sources of Information about Diet

Here is the best information about dietary therapy that we can offer at this time, and it is actually a lot. Additional information will surely be available as this theory is tested and developed over time. Further experience and testing these ideas will result in some being abandoned and others expanded. As a consequence of more work and better understanding, results should improve. This information is offered for your consideration and review as an educational opportunity. None of this is intended to replace direct treatment you are receiving from your personal physician.

After considerable discussion, we decided it is not necessary to explain the huge body of ancient Traditional Chinese Medicine (TCM) knowledge that is the foundation of our theory for the dietary treatment of PD. It could easily require several large textbooks to explain all of the necessary TCM principles and concepts fully, and that might not be adequate. We concluded, most people do not really care about the ancient theory and principles of TCM. Most just want the basic information about what to eat and what not to eat. Those who really want to gain a foundation of understanding in TCM necessary to make sense of this information should simply contact **PDI** for the needed resources for independent TCM study.

How They Did It

All the men who report greatest success with their PD have done more than just follow the dietary changes we suggested for them. Sorry, dietary changes alone will not do it. They were also following an Alternative Medicine therapy plan from the **PDI** web site, taking several different types of vitamins and systemic enzymes while they were also following the PD diet.

The scientists who are reading this last paragraph are in a tizzy. They are holding their heads saying, "You can't do that! That is not good research! You must not allow those men to do anything else to treat their PD while they are following the diet program. How will you know which one of these two basic approaches is actually helping these people? This is not good science!" And, of course, they would be right. This is not good science. That's OK.

Frankly, **PDI** does not at this time subscribe to the true research approach that must be eventually taken. Currently **PDI** and the men we consult with are more interested in what is know as "doing what you have to do to get over PD." It is our opinion that we will continue for a while longer improving this "shotgun" approach to treating PD. We feel that we have so much more work to do in this area that there is no good way to limit the scope of care to just a few people. We will attempt to bring as many cases along to success as possible, then determine retroactively how the various strategies worked. Our survey information and our research studies are not complete, and perhaps will never be complete to the satisfaction of the strict research scientists. We are more interested in helping PD victims; the research will work itself out later.

This is an extremely important point, because it shows that you must treat your PD from several different directions at the same time; this is part of the synergy that is stressed so much in all the **PDI** information about treating PD. This is a difficult problem to treat, and takes considerable effort for success. Small efforts are usually unsuccessful. If you feel like doing just a little, then expect to get similar results – just a little.

The important thing to remember is that from our best information, diet therapy alone by avoidance or addition will not get the job done: You must also use the vitamins, enzymes and different therapies as found on the **PDI** web site. Go to www.peyronies-disease-help.com

Practical Suggestions for Dietary Changes

In the real world not many men have easy or frequent access to kohlrabi, aduki beans, alfalfa, or pumpkin. Probably you only eat pumpkin in a pie once or twice a year around Thanksgiving. Do not let that bother you. You will see many other foods can be included into your diet for variety and good taste. However, if you are a big fan of aduki beans and you happen to eat a lot of pumpkin, be our guest and make those two a major part of your diet.

The idea with the foods on the "Add" list is to find those that you already eat and enjoy, that are easy and convenient to eat. Make them a larger part of your daily food intake than you usually do. It is not necessary to eat all of these foods on the "Add" list. Just emphasize as often as possible, those foods on this list you already eat and enjoy.

If you cannot eat many foods from the "Add" list on a particular day, then definitely follow the "Avoid" list closely – very closely. Do not get the wrong idea: The "Add" list is important and you should work with it, but the "Avoid" list is perhaps even more important. Use both the "Avoid" and "Add" lists, but if you cannot get any of the "Add" foods into your diet one day, PLEASE follow the "Avoid" list, because it is so important.

Make a sincere effort to go out of your way to actually add these foods into your diet, especially if you eat at Chinese or Thai restaurants. This would be a good excuse for the next few weeks to go to these restaurants more often if you can. Don't whine and make excuses, just do it. If you go to McDonald's four times a week or your favorite Italian restaurant once a week, why not go for a while to the Thai restaurant instead?

Explain to your wife what you are trying to do. Talk to her. Give her this book to read. She needs to know what you are going to do, and definitely ask her to read this chapter.

Foods to Avoid in your PD Diet Therapy Plan

Avoid cold foods and drinks – Don't put cold things into your body.

No ice in drinks – ask the waitress for water with no ice.

No cold food from the refrigerator.

Ideally food and drink should be at room temperature or warm.

If you don't like taste of Coke at room temperature, then just don't drink it.

Avoid all dairy products – Doubly-to-be-avoided as they are consumed cold.

Ice cream, cheese, milk, butter, sour cream, yogurt, kefir

Don't forget about foods that contain cheese or milk ingredients
Pizza
Pancakes
Salad dressings made with sour cream
Cream in you coffee
Butter on toast
Shredded cheese that restaurants put on salads these days – remove it

Many dairy products can be consumed in an average day, because they are often hidden among other ingredients.

If you must have a bowl of cereal for breakfast, try goat's milk – but don't forget to take the chill out of it.

Homogenized milk contains xanthine oxidase, a milk enzyme that is normally found only in the liver of humans, but is in high concentration in the palmar connective tissue of patients with Dupuytren's contracture and other conditions in which the inactivation of nitric oxide is an important factor (such as Peyronie's disease). This is another good reason to avoid milk if you have PD.

Avoid alcoholic drinks

Beer, wine, whiskey, etc.

Avoid foods on this list

Meat in general, but definitely all greasy and fatty meat – You do not have to become a vegetarian, but definitely cut back on eating red meat – the further the better. A simple strategy is to eat meat at 50% fewer meals; half of your meals should be meatless initially. After you are comfortable eating meat less often, then eat smaller portions of meat when you do eat it. Go for quality of meat, not quantity. The worse kind of meat is processed meat like sausage (fatty and greasy) and any meats that do not have to be refrigerated.

Eggs – Same as for milk; we eat more than we realize as an ingredient.

Mushrooms

Soy products (tofu, soy milk)

Bananas

Salt – avoid completely, or at least cut it way back

Foods to Add to your PD Diet Therapy Plan

Add these foods to the diet as often as possible

Aduki beans

Alfalfa

Almonds

Apricot

Asparagus

Broccoli

Cabbage

Carrot

Cherry

Citrus peel

Celery

Chickpeas (garbanzo beans) – used to make hummus; add cayenne peppers for a good kick: hummus is available in many regular grocery stores. Hummus is really a great food, try it!

Chives

Cucumber

Date – not a bad desert, or substitute for the usual candy and junk foods we eat; get a pack of it, and you might be surprised

Eggplant

Fig – not a bad desert, or substitute for the usual candy and junk foods we eat; get a pack of it, and you might be surprised

Kohlrabi

Leek

Lettuce

Mustard Green

Navy beans – vegetarian navy bean soup should include many vegetables from this list

Onion

Orange

Papaya

Parsley

Parsnip

Pears

Peas

Pineapple

Pumpkin

Radish

Rutabaga

Scallion – this is the long green onions that are so popular in Asian cooking; when you go to the Chinese restaurant, ask for more of these than they usually include in whatever you order

Spinach – grocery stores now have it available in prepared bags

Squash

Strawberry

Sweet potato – bake them like white potatoes

Turnips – can be substituted for potatoes when you want to eat mashed potatoes; just peel, cube, boil and mash like a potato

Vinegar – found in many salad dressings, mustard, coleslaw, etc.

Add these Bitter herbs and hot spices

Black pepper

Basil – very popular at Thai and Italian restaurants – eat in these restaurants more often for the next few weeks

Cayenne – buy a bottle of it and sprinkle a little on different foods

Cardamom

Chamomile tea – drink one or two cups of this tea a day

Chaparral

Cinnamon

Ginger – ask for dishes with a lot of this at Thai or Chinese restaurants

Nutmeg

Pau d'arco

Peach seed (can be ordered from **PDI** in capsule form)

Spearmint tea – drink one or two cups of this tea a day

Rosemary

Turmeric (can be ordered from **PDI** in capsule form)

Valerian – drink one or two cups of this tea a day (can be ordered from **PDI** in capsule form)

Talk to Your Cook

Ask the cook in the family (probably your wife) to read this chapter, if not the whole book. Ask her to help you change your diet for the next several weeks. Show her you are sincere in changing your diet to help your PD.

Do not expect her to go out of her way looking for special recipes that feature foods on the "Add" list, if you eat all wrong when you are away from home. So, when you eat your lunch away from home, you cannot eat a greasy cheeseburger or pizza and wash it down with a cold beer. You must be as dedicated to this project, as you expect her to be dedicated to your success.

Warning; If you are the kind of guy who cannot eat a lot of hot spicy food, then do not do it. Skip the cayenne pepper and eat more of other foods you can comfortably handle.

- **If it turns out there are only three or four foods on the "Add" list that you really like, and you can eat them without a lot of special effort on your part or your wife's part, then those are the ones to emphasize in your diet. Don't make this a painful or hard thing to do, but, definitely do what you can and stay with it.**

At the end of this chapter you will find a simple list titled "Add and Avoid." Copy this list for the next time you go shopping. Check off those foods you want to stress in your diet. You surely do not have to eat all of those on the "Add" list; just significantly increase those that appeal to you. Conversely, it would be good at least to eat a minimal amount of those foods on the "Avoid" list or eliminate them all together if you can.

Chew your food very thoroughly

Slow down when you eat; chew your food well. This is a very important part of the program.

There are several good health reasons to chew your food well. The first has simply to do with absorption of nutrients and enzymes. The others have to do with Traditional Chinese Medicine principles of energy absorption and movement of chi energy.

Each time you sit down to eat, remind yourself that you must slow the pace of eating. Chew your food more completely than ever before. You should chew your food so completely that little conscious effort is needed to swallow it, since your food should be so finely broken down and liquefied that it just slides down your throat.

From our survey we find that many men with PD have digestive problems. This is an issue of interest to anyone with PD. The intent of asking you to chew your food thoroughly is first to directly assist your PD, but it will likely also improve your digestion and elimination. Do not misunderstand, within Traditional Chinese Medicine a direct connection is found between eating of food that is incompletely chewed and a wide variety of health problems, like PD. The purpose of this request is specifically for PD, but it could also benefit the many common digestive complaints of these same men.

It can be difficult at first to simply take more time to chew each mouthful of food. You might feel like you are wasting time, or perhaps as though people are watching you eat in some bizarre way, or they are actually aware of how long you are chewing your food. Get over it; no one is looking and no one cares that you are chewing longer than the average person.

Lifelong daily habits of this nature are difficult to break. Expect to forget and lapse often when you start chewing longer. You can do it. You can make this very fundamental change in your daily way of eating. It is a very important part of the dietary treatment of PD; do not make the mistake of thinking you should skip it.

That is all there is to it. It is simple on one hand, and as difficult as leaving your comfort zone on the other hand. The ease of following through with any PD treatment is related to how serious you are about getting your life back together. To a mind that is truly made up and focused on victory over PD, this little experiment with eating differently for a few weeks is never a big deal. If you are not comfortable with the idea of these changes, then you must reconsider how comfortable you are in having PD.

Again, diet is very important in treating PD, but so are the various enzymes and vitamins that are key in making this program work for you. Check it out on the **PDI** web site.

It is **PDI**'s opinion that a major piece of the PD puzzle could fall into place when the cause of the sporadic scar changes is discovered. It is our current opinion that the reason so many men experience slight frequent changes in their PD scar is because of the usual daily changes and fluctuations in the diet. Some days a man might accidentally eat more foods on the avoid list and his scar gets worse, and some days he might accidentally eat no food on the avoid list and his scar gets smaller and softer.

Once the phenomenon of the variable PD scar is better understood, we all could be much closer to a real "cure" to this problem.

Shopping List – copy and take with you

"Avoid":

- ☐ Cold drinks and foods
- ☐ Dairy - Ice cream, cheese, milk, butter, sour cream, yogurt, kefir
- ☐ Alcoholic drinks
- ☐ Meat in general – 50% less meat than usual; only lean meat
- ☐ Eggs
- ☐ Mushrooms
- ☐ Soy products (tofu, soy milk)
- ☐ Bananas
- ☐ Salt

"Add" as much as possible:

- ☐ Aduki beans
- ☐ Alfalfa
- ☐ Almonds
- ☐ Apricot
- ☐ Asparagus
- ☐ Black pepper
- ☐ Broccoli
- ☐ Cabbage
- ☐ Carrot
- ☐ Cherry
- ☐ Citrus peel
- ☐ Celery
- ☐ Chickpeas (garbanzo beans)

- ☐ Chives
- ☐ Cucumber
- ☐ Date
- ☐ Eggplant
- ☐ Fig
- ☐ Kohlrabi
- ☐ Leek
- ☐ Lettuce
- ☐ Mustard Green
- ☐ Navy beans
- ☐ Onion
- ☐ Orange
- ☐ Papaya
- ☐ Parsley

- ☐ Parsnip
- ☐ Pears
- ☐ Peas
- ☐ Pineapple
- ☐ Pumpkin
- ☐ Radish
- ☐ Rutabaga
- ☐ Scallion
- ☐ Spinach
- ☐ Squash
- ☐ Strawberry
- ☐ Sweet potato
- ☐ Turnips
- ☐ Vinegar

Bitter herbs and hot spices:

- ☐ Basil
- ☐ Cayenne
- ☐ Cardamom
- ☐ Chamomile tea
- ☐ Chaparral

- ☐ Cinnamon
- ☐ Ginger
- ☐ Nutmeg
- ☐ Pau d'arco
- ☐ Peach seed

- ☐ Spearmint tea
- ☐ Rosemary
- ☐ Turmeric
- ☐ Valerian

Chapter 6 – Improve Your Life in Spite of PD

Ω **- To live a better life, be happier and healthier in spite of your PD, and increase your chance of successfully treating it ...**

... you must determine if you are doing things during the course of your average day – simple and common things – that could be stressing and irritating the PD scar. This takes some close review and observation of your actions and habits. Once you have determined that you have been guilty of stressing your PD, then it is further necessary to change what are probably lifelong habits. Sound like a major project? It could be, but it could also be another important step toward success over your PD. Allow this chapter to guide you through this process of discovery and change.

All day long I communicate with men who have PD. I find even after they have seen their family doctor and/or urologist several times, and have perhaps lived with this disease for years, they still do not understand their problem. It is apparent they have neither been given information about the most fundamental and important aspects of living with this problem, nor have they figured out much on their own. Since they do not know much about their condition, they might continually do many things that could frequently aggravate or re-injure their PD.

Sometimes I wonder if the actual difference between those men whose PD just goes away on its own, and those whose PD lasts is simply a lifetime of being guilty of small daily re-injury, or not. Interesting concept, isn't it?

This chapter presents helpful advice to make living with PD safer and easier, discussing common and simple activities that perhaps you should be doing differently because you have PD. By modifying some of these frequent daily activities, you should be reducing stress on your scar and avoiding re-injury to the susceptible tissue that has already been traumatized. It is the goal of this chapter to increase the odds that you might recover from your PD.

Most of the advice found in this chapter, and even this entire book, is based primarily on common sense, and direct observations, guided by what we currently consider to be true about PD from the available scientific information. Actually, no one knows much for certain about this problem known as Peyronie's disease. This information, presented for your education and consideration, is compiled from the current pool of scientific knowledge and a large dose of common sense. Many of these ideas come from talking with and emailing to men who are in a variety of bad PD circumstances. Any or all of it might change at any time, since **PDI** receives an ongoing stream of information every day from people just like you.

Hush-hush

A great degree of awkwardness and discomfort is displayed in current society when discussing the penis and what it does. The idea that some personal things are better left unspoken is often true, and represents good manners, but not when it comes to learning about life with PD.

We have to delve into many private areas of personal behavior and private habits if this is to be a useful and practical source of information for PD readers. Unless a certain level of honesty and frankness is used, the effectiveness of this communication and the completeness of your understanding will be reduced.

Since the subject of PD concerns a disease of the penis, and the penis is essentially used in two basic functions – sexual activity and urinary elimination – most of the topics discussed in this book are often considered to be of a personal 'hush-hush" nature. Perhaps that is just because I am an American and most men with whom I communicate are also Americans. It is said that Europeans are far more open and honest – even blunt – in all these areas. Nonetheless, most discussion in this chapter will cover topics that are usually not spoken of, and a few that are often not even thought about.

Not Rocket Science

Many subjects, when taken down to their essence, become surprisingly simple and self-evident. In this rather basic form, many ideas seem almost too obvious and not worth mentioning. It seems that surely everyone must be aware of a basic truth when it is sitting plainly in front of the reader. It is almost embarrassing to discuss the obvious, and many topics discussed here are taken to the point of being that obvious.

None of the following is rocket science, but might as well be since it is rare for anyone to think or know much about some of these topics. Most men seem to be oblivious to these little **PDI** gems of information and insight.

Simply stated, most of this advice centers around two very fundamental and painfully obvious principles for living with PD. These two concepts, when followed to their logical conclusion during real life activities, will most definitely have a favorable influence on the course of your PD recovery:

- Do not injure your penis further than it is already.
- Promote good blood circulation to the lower pelvis.

Pretty obvious, isn't it? But how you go about <u>doing</u> these two things can be complex and not commonly known or considered.

The rest of this chapter will expand upon these two simple rules, or will be spent describing different ways of applying these two rules to your life as a PD sufferer.

Protect and Take Care of Your Injured Penis

Keep in mind that if you have PD, it could have started when your penis received a small or large injury in a direct or indirect way. According to current thinking and belief, if you are genetically predisposed to PD it is possible the trauma was so minor that you did not even notice it at the time. If you are not genetically predisposed the trauma was probably greater. It does not really matter how little or how much trauma was involved. In response, the penis overreacted at the site of injury by producing excessive scar tissue. Even though this may have happened some time ago, the penis continues to harbor tissue that is foreign to the area it is in. The presence of this foreign tissue has altered the elasticity of the thin but tough internal membranes of the penis, and interfered with the ability of the blood vessels to close when attempting to create an erection. As a result of this foreign scar tissue, four classic findings of PD develop:

1. A nodule, a bump, a lump, a bead, a ribbon, or a cord of fibrous tissue develops within the thin membrane of the penis called the tunica albuginea. This growth is usually referred to as a scar or plaque. Oftentimes, it is the first thing detected to announce the presence of the disease. In some men the scar or nodule is merely difficult to locate. In others, even their doctors are unable to locate the scar or nodule, although all other signs and findings are present to make a diagnosis.

2. One or more bends or curvatures of the penis develop during an erection, which were not present before the PD started.

3. Reduced ability to achieve a full hard erection as you did prior to the onset of PD; sometimes only minor softness develops. At other times it is totally flaccid or soft. The reduced ability to achieve erection can affect just part of the penis (the part farthest from the abdomen, or closest to the head of the penis), and other times it can affect the entire penis, resulting in total impotency.

4. Pain of variable location and intensity. For some the pain is constant, in others the pain occurs only during erection, and still others only when non-erect. The pain intensity can range from minor to intense.

The presence of this foreign scar tissue creates a state of instability to the structural and functional integrity of the penis, perpetuated by ongoing and continual re-injury. This is a critical point. Think of the scar as a thorn in the side of the penis. The scar makes the penis feel and work differently. It makes all penile tissue more vulnerable to continual irritation and re-injury from actions, pressure and situations that were too minor prior to PD to have any impact on the penis.

With the onset of PD, it seems as though everything in your life changes. The tissue sensitivity created by the presence of scar material causes the penis is more vulnerable to everyday stresses that previously were easily tolerated.

Few people would consider using some of these strategies if they had no penile problem. However, given that life is different when you have PD, these are necessary and useful strategies to offer protection from ongoing re-injury and increase the chances of recovery.

What Not to Do

Here is a brief discussion of what not to do, to avoid additional injury to your penis. This is a broad collection of common sense ideas that are not all that common, unfortunately. They have been collected and developed over time through the direct experience of many men with PD. Many are little more than common sense and simple observations that usually go unnoticed.

They all can be grouped under the heading of "Don't be your own worse enemy."

Big Idea: DO NOT GET ROUGH WITH YOUR PENIS – EVEN IF NOT ERECT

Men understand that the nature of the genital tissue is rather delicate and can evoke considerable and disproportionate levels of pain if abused.

1. **Do not avoid sexual activity**. Sexual activity is therapeutic in general for healthy people, and men with PD in particular, because it does increase local circulation to the lower pelvis. In addition, it will generally reduce the occurrence of the extreme depression and anger that so many men with PD go through. Sexual expression is a large measure of what makes us human. When denied by illness, the need to engage in this intimate level of communication with someone we care deeply about does not stop. Loss of the sexual aspect of life can be devastating to the mental and physical well-being of either or both partners, and their life together.

   The only limitation or caution is, do not engage in sexual activity in such a way that you could injure yourself further. Go slowly, easily, cautiously and with some thought, asking yourself if a particular activity may put you at risk of stressing the penile tissue. Basically, it comes down to enjoy yourself, but be careful.

2. **Do not bend an erection.** When erect the penis forms a very rigid cylinder hence the nickname for the erect penis, "boner." However, during an erection the layered or laminated tissues of the penis are very vulnerable to injury. This is the reason many men who actually remember a specific injury to the penis will often report that the injury involved a sudden and forceful bending of the penis while it was erect. As a cautionary note, this makes intercourse a time of potential danger since the pubic bone or inner thigh of the sexual partner can be rammed against the penis, causing a painful and sudden bend.

The erect penis is vulnerable anywhere along the length of the shaft from the base of the penis, at the attachment near the pubic bone, and at any point along the shaft, up to and including the head or glans.

3. **Do not stress the penis during sex play**. Do not play that famous game of tucking your penis between legs and hiding it from your wife during sex play. Do not force an erection into unnatural positions. Do not allow your penis to be aggressively handled while erect. If she gets wild and carried away, it is up you – the owner of the penis, who will suffer – to remain sober and vigilant that no harm comes to you. Do not get crazy during sex.

4. **Do not use a "cock ring."** A cock ring is a small diameter rubber ring device that is slipped over the erection in an effort to trap blood and sustain the erect state longer than usual. It works on the penis very much in the way a tourniquet traps blood in an arm or leg. And just like a tourniquet, problems can occur if the blood circulation is stopped too long or too well. This can lead to damage and injury not only to the area of the penis that sustained the prolonged pressure, but also to all the membranes and internal tissues of the entire penis. These tissues can sustain injury from anoxia (lack of oxygen) by denying the necessary oxygen that all parts of the body require.

5. **Do not cross your legs improperly.** Do not sit with your legs crossed in such a way that brings the inner thighs tightly together and thus pushes and presses on the genitals. There are two ways you should not cross your legs.

   A. **Usually described as crossing your legs "like a woman."** Women will cross their legs by placing the back of one knee on top of the knee cap of the other, in a very tight overlapping arrangement. For men, because of their cargo in the crotch, this exerts pressure on the genitals resulting in reduced blood and lymphatic circulation to the entire groin region. For the entire pelvic region to be healthy, even the prostate gland, do nothing that reduces the circulation in your groin.

   B. **Crossing your legs at the ankles.** Described as laying one ankle over the other ankle while the legs are held out straight. This technique compresses the genitals also, and should also be avoided.

If you must cross your legs do it in that very manly fashion that is not very polite. It is not polite because it most definitely causes a widening of the space between the legs, the crotch, and a display of the groin region. This is described as sitting with one ankle laying on top of the knee of the other leg. The top leg that is doing the crossing is allowed to roll outward and lay horizontally, creating a wide angle or "V" at the crotch. This opens the space between the legs, and applies very little compression to reduce circulation. If you must cross your legs when you sit, do it this way.

6. **Do not wear tight clothing**. If you become erect while wearing tight fitting clothes, stress to the penis will definitely occur when it happens that the penis has no where for it to expand and lengthen when erect. Thus, avoid wearing tight fitting traditional "Jockey-type" white underwear that holds genitals close to body. The same goes for tight jeans.

7. **Do not apply force or pressure directly to the scar or to the penis** – don't rub or massage the scar, since this might further injure the thin tunica albuginea. If your injury was so minimal that you do not remember it, imagine what could happen if you apply repeated and/or prolonged direct force to this area.

8. **Do not become discouraged.** Stay as positive as possible and do not lose sight of the fact that many men experience total and complete remission of their PD for no apparent reason. If PD can leave without treatment, then why not you? Are the men whose PD just disappears simply lucky, or did they do something important accidentally that helped their problem to recover? If some men get lucky by accident, can you also get lucky if you try to do many things correctly to heal and repair the damaged tissue of the penis?

   If PD can leave without treatment and if PD can get worse with treatment, then this only proves the great void of knowledge for what we know about PD or its treatment. Think what might happen for you if you become healthier and better able to heal and repair yourself by spending some time working to improve the function of your immune response.

What to Do

Next is a longer discussion of what you should do during the course of your day as a PD sufferer. This discussion was developed from the observations, common sense ideas and experiences of many men who have lived with PD for many years. It is offered to you for your consideration as an educational experience and a chance to develop a better understanding of the relationship between what you do and how your body responds.

Improve Your Attitude about PD

Through my daily communication with men who have PD, and as someone who had an active case of PD for a little more than two years, I have made an observation about the attitude of men with PD. This observation is that the great percent of men with PD seem to dissociate themselves from their penis as if it were "the enemy." In many ways they express themselves as though their penis is now somehow foreign to them, detached in some way, no longer a part of them although it is still attached in the same place it was always found. Their attitude is one of rejection and hostility to this previously friendly body part. They express in many ways an attitude that their penis has turned against them and is now the ugly enemy that causes pain and is no longer pleasurable. They seem not to think in terms of PD being a health problem that needs help, but just a bad situation they are in that has caused their penis to work incorrectly.

PD is the enemy. Your penis is not the enemy. Don't get confused on this issue.

Perhaps this attitude is the result of reading all the negative and hopeless opinions about PD; perhaps it is how men react when the medical profession is not keen on doing anything but advocating surgical procedures that often leave a man further scarred and more impotent than before the surgery.

A more realistic, honest and constructive attitude is based on the idea that the body can and does heal when given the opportunity, even with a condition as stubborn as PD.

Does that sound like heresy? Does that sound like quackery? Does that sound like the evil voodoo that all the guys warn about on the PD forums? Well maybe that is how it sounds to you. If the thought that PD can be healed by the body strikes you as uncomfortably wrong, then you are probably a very good medical patient who believes the standard medical approach to this problem.

It is my experience that good medical patients do not know much about their problem. They merely rely on their medical doctor to take care of them. They turn their problem over to their doctor, to let him worry about it, and they do not ask many questions or get involved much in the treatment of their problem. Even if you are a true believer in everything that your medical doctor tells you, another viewpoint becomes apparent with just a little independent thinking about PD.

Medical literature emphatically states, "There is no such thing as a medical cure for PD." Yet, in another statement from the standard medical literature you will also find, "PD just disappears in 5-50% of the cases within the first 18 months. For those remaining individuals in whom PD does not disappear by itself, it is permanent." What these statements are saying is, "PD is permanent unless your body heals it on its own, without medical intervention. We do not know how it happens, but it happens about half the time."

This statement comes down to the failure of organized medicine to understand the problem of PD, and the supremacy of the body to heal in 50% of PD cases.

All opinions and statements about PD that come from within the practice of medicine are held to be true. The medical researchers acknowledge that the body is successful about half of the time in correcting PD, yet the method and process of the body's success in healing PD seem never to be investigated. The direction of a cure for PD is focused by <u>medical</u> researches who continue to look vainly for a <u>medical</u> solution to this problem. It never seems to occur to these researches that the answer is already active and in place in the 5-50% of men whose PD disappears by itself. The answer to healing PD is to be found somewhere in being more like members of that "lucky" 5-50% group.

Along this line of thought, my good friend, Jim Leahy, once wrote to me, "If the medical professionals feel the body heals PD in about 50% of the cases, isn't that a good reason to do all you can to help your body do its job? Isn't that a good reason to put a lot of the natural supplements to work in the body as recommend in the **PDI** therapy program? It sounds to me like the medical professionals are really showing their lack of understanding how the body works when they say, 'let the body heal your PD, but don't give it any help.' They are contradicting themselves by telling us on one hand, take care for your body, eat healthy, get rest, drink lots of fluids, take your vitamin E.... but, on the other hand, don't do anything natural for your PD." Yes, I think Jim really has it right.

We all know that the medical profession advocates all of these simple and logical health measures for other health problems, they just don't seem to apply it to PD. The **PDI** approach to this problem is simply based on these common health recommendations from the medical profession.

If you wish to explore this line of thought further, please go to the **PDI** web site and click on the links for "Treatment Options" and "Philosophy." There you will learn how to increase your chance of getting healthier and increase your chance of healing this terrible disease. With a better understanding of what you can and should do to try to help yourself out of the PD predicament, your attitude about your PD will improve. It will help you have a different – and better – attitude than you have had since that fateful day you first heard about Peyronie's disease.

Warm it up

Use moist heat on you penis if you are going to be doing any kind of external therapy. For that matter, even if all you are doing are internal therapies of vitamins, minerals and enzymes, moist heat is still a good inexpensive therapy to do every day, all by itself.

Moist heat applied before other therapies (DMSO, vitamin E oil) will give you an extra advantage. If you precede most any external therapy (or sexual activity) with moist heat you will bring extra blood to the genital area. The additional blood flow and increased lymphatic drainage that will result from the application of this heat, will allow other therapies to penetrate deeper and expand the tissue more fully. In addition you can also apply more moist heat after any or all of your therapies. Moist heat will assure a better therapeutic response.

A hot shower is generally not effective because the heat is applied in such a broad area, that additional blood cannot be sent over the entire surface. You will not experience the degree of increased blood flow and lymphatic drainage as when the heat is focused to a smaller and more specific area.

To apply moist heat to your genital area, first cover the surface that you will be laying on to keep the area dry. Prepare three towels.

The first is used to cover the surface that you will be sitting or laying on.

The second should be a large clean towel. Soak it water as hot as you can stand to handle. Wring the towel out as completely as possible so that it is not dripping excess water. Lie down in a comfortable position. Apply the large hot moist towel to the genital area for 5-15 minutes, with special attention to covering and wrapping specifically around the penis, being careful not to burn yourself.

The third is a towel to cover and insulate the moist towel to keep it as hot as you can stand, for as long as possible.

The first time you do this, PLEASE check yourself after the first five minutes and check yourself again five minutes after the first check, to assure that you are not burning your tender genital tissue. If it should happen, because that is the nature of accidents, use:

1. **Ice pack to the area** for 20 minutes only, no more. After 20 minutes the response of the body to the ice changes, and the tissue begins to swell and favor retention of inflammatory by-products. Do this twice the first day and then daily until you are no longer in pain.

2. **Neosporin topical ointment** applied to the area of injury according to package instructions. Keep the area clean and covered with sterile gauze.

3. **Aloe vera gel** applied to the area will speed healing.

4. **Determine what you did wrong with the heat; don't do it again**, because you will be using moist heat again in a slightly different manner, as it is still a good thing to do. Adjust and modify your technique so you will not burn yourself again.

At the conclusion of using the moist heat application you should be nicely pink – only. Not red. You should not feel like you are sore to the touch after using the hot towel. If possible, keep the hot moist towel in place while doing other therapy; apply moist heat while doing DMSO, vitamin E oil and copper peptide treatment, or soft tissue massage to the lower pelvis.

As a very effective option, you can also simply use a hot water bottle wrapped with a moist towel to the genital when you go to bed, or simply put it in place if you will be sitting for a long time in front of the TV, your computer or even your car. Or, you can even put a half or full cup of rice in an old sock, tie off the open end, and heat it in the microwave for a few minutes. This is an easy and inexpensive way to make a handy reusable heating method for your problem area. Every little bit helps.

Do not underestimate the value of heat applied to the penis to speed up healing – it might seem old-fashioned, but it works wonders. Do it!

Self-treatment of PD

Since men experience a spontaneous recovery from PD in an estimated 5-50% of cases (depending on the study you read), it would be good to attempt to be as much like those lucky men as possible. Unfortunately, they are a difficult group to communicate with since once a person is rid of the disease, he stops reading and communicating about it with others who still have it.

With limited data from the men who experience spontaneous recovery, we are only left to speculate how they get over their PD in some as yet unknown way. They must be healthier, stronger or functioning better than the men who do not repair and heal their PD. When we understand what makes them so different in the important way they self-correct their PD, we will have a better way to approach PD treatment. Until then, the current **PDI** concept appears to be the best and most logical course of action to overcome this distressing condition. This is the prime area of interest for anyone who has PD: "What is different between me and the guy whose PD goes away by itself?" The short answer is, no one knows for sure. The longer answer is, there are some very good ideas that make sense and are backed up by sufficient scientific research. One of the basic ideas behind a good self-directed PD therapy plan is that it should increase the immune response to injury. For a much greater look into that area of Alternative Medicine please go to the **PDI** web site, at www.peyronies-disease-help.com. Go to the Treatment Options section for a long and detailed discussion of possible therapy choices that might apply to your situation.

In that larger section you will find many different potential therapies to consider. The one concept behind it all is the greater the number of therapies you have working together simultaneously, the greater your chances of increasing your ability to self-repair the PD scar. As you will find in the **PDI** web site, this is the power of synergy; the combining of several smaller forces so that they have a greater total effect than if they were taken alone. It can be explained in the simple example of "1+1+1 = 5." This is the power of synergy. We recommend anyone with PD attempt to use synergy to harness the ability to heal and repair like the lucky 5-50% group of men who healed their own PD.

The **PDI** web site is huge, about 175 pages, and growing, including all levels of information concerning the subject of PD. Special emphasis is directed to the Alternative Medicine treatment of this condition, with massive and aggressive use of many conservative therapies in an effort to increase the body's ability to repair and heal the PD scar. There is no need to highlight or repeat what is on that web site, since it is freely available to all who wish to investigate this topic for themselves.

"Sit down, Mr. President, make yourself comfortable"

No, this is not a polite gesture to a politician. I am suggesting you do something that has really made a huge difference to men with PD.

It seems that men with PD, either before they develop the condition or perhaps just because they have the condition, can become very uncomfortable in the genitals and crotch after sitting for any length of time. When sitting they notice that the entire genital area becomes pressed and bound up by the seam at the crotch of the pants in such a way that is most genuinely uncomfortable. But even more important than the personal distress that it causes, it is my contention that this pressure is very bad for PD because of the reduced blood and lymphatic circulation it causes. To be so tied up and strangled by pants seams and zippers that the area can go numb after a while, cannot be healthy for the scrotum, testicles and penis.

Actually, none of this discussion is about comfort. You will certainly feel more comfortable when you create more space in the crotch of your pants, and in so doing reposition your genitals. However, that is not why you should do it. You should do it, as someone with PD, because the pressure that is causing the discomfort is severely restricting blood and lymphatic flow in that area. And that, sir, is not good. You want good circulation in your genitals and you want to be more mindful of this need from now on.

You must come to understand it would be good for your PD to create a habit of making more room for yourself when you go to sit down for any length of time. Once you do, you find you have been unnecessarily tolerating that dull aching and deep pressure in your crotch for so many years even though it is so easy to eliminate. You will wonder why you have not taken better care of yourself sooner. It is a good habit to develop, because it will assure better blood flow in and out and better lymphatic drainage of the genitals. And this is, as Martha Stewart would say, "a good thing."

Here is a little story to explain this point. President Lyndon Johnson was a decisive man of action, a crafty and aggressive politician who knew how to take total control of any situation that was important to him. And apparently his "comfort" was very important to him. Your comfort is even more important because it tells you a lot about the circulation that is so important to your PD.

68

Many years after his death the thousands of hours of tape recordings of his various activities, great and not so great, were made public. This discussion concerns a very funny tape recording made of his conversation in the Oval Office of the White House, as he was being fitted for six pair of new pants. President Johnson did not care that the entire event was being tape recorded. It was the summer of 1964 and the Viet Nam war was not going well. Yet, his interest in the comfort of his "nuts" was very keen and was being documented on a tape recording for posterity.

Lyndon Baines Johnson had been president for only about nine months, though he had already signed the Civil Rights Act, accelerated the war in Vietnam, and watched entire neighborhoods in Harlem go up in smoke. Even so, on August 11, 1964, Johnson telephoned Joe Haggar, his personal tailor, from the Oval Office and said, "If you don't want me running around the White House naked, you better get me some clothes."

In his slow Southern drawl, the most powerful man in the world then proceeded to give very specific instructions to this tailor that he wanted to be "comfortable" when he sat for a long time.

He described in detail how he wanted each of the six new pairs of pants made to his specifications. We learn from the tape recording, "Now, another thing, the crotch, down where your nuts hang, it's always a little too tight," said Johnson. "So when you make them up, give me an inch where I can let it out there, because they cut me. They're just like riding a wire fence."

He described it perfectly, didn't he? "Like riding a wire fence" really explains it well. And just because it can be such a problem for the men with PD, let us now address this topic of "presidential" importance.

Give Yourself Extra Room Down There

If you are already sitting, and you can not or do not want to get up, you need to create more room for your "comfort" without making a display of yourself. Ideally you would want to be in a private situation when you do this, as in your car or your own home.

Actually, we have all seen many baseball players frequently pull and tug and stretch the cloth material around their crotch while they are on the playing field. They take great effort to reposition themselves in this most private way while out in public – with millions of people watching, no less. Any man with PD should not be too shy about taking care of his personal comfort and well-being. Here is how:

1. Prepare yourself and your groin when you are getting ready to sit in a large overstuffed chair or sofa.

2. Simply pinch the cloth (Careful: do not pinch more than that!) below the bottom of the zipper. Give it a nice downward and forward pull so that the twisted and wrinkled material in that area is straightened out, making more room for your genitals. If you do it fast and nonchalantly no one will notice, or at least be unsure that you even did it.

3. With your pants so arranged and more room available down there, you will be able to sit in far greater comfort with minimal reduction of blood flow to the genitals.

Here is an alternate method, if you find that you are getting squashed and uncomfortable while you are already sitting.

1. While sitting, firmly place both feet on the floor and push your upper back against the backrest of the chair you are sitting on. As you do this, slightly arch your back and lift your butt off the seat of the chair. Almost all pressure and contact will be exerted on the feet and upper back. Your butt and the back of your thighs should be off the chair.

2. You are now free to reach down to the crotch of your pants and pull the material down and away from your genitals. You will feel an immediate sense of freedom and room. Now, you will be just as the comfortable as any President ever was.

While you will note an unusual sense of comfort and freedom from pressure and restriction, this maneuver is not only about how it feels to create that extra space, but more so to reduce pressure and restriction on the genitals.

Get in the habit of tending to yourself this way to assure you have good blood circulation at all times. This little application of tender loving care is very important to the healing process.

Consider having a tailor "lower the crotch" in your pants by an inch or two. It will not affect the way the pants fit otherwise. Cost should not be much more than $10-15 each.

Sleep Like a Log – But the Correct Way

Throughout life, men get erections during the night (nocturnal erections), that have nothing to do with direct sexual arousal. In fact, the great majority of these erections go unnoticed because the erection occurs while the man is in deep slumber.

Sleep studies over the past 40 years have established that all normal and healthy males from birth to death have erections of a certain intensity and rigidity, lasting fifteen to thirty minutes, roughly every ninety minutes all night long. These erections coincide with rapid eye movement (REM) sleep. The occurrence of REM sleep, a specific phase of sleep, can be influenced by drugs, depression and sleep disorders such as apnea, resulting in a lack of nocturnal erections.

Current information suggests that nocturnal erections occur for the maintenance of the cavernous (spongy) tissue in the penis. The cavernous tissue, responsible for the engorgement and enlargement of the penis that occurs during an erection, is saturated with oxygen during an erection. Thus, nocturnal erections are a necessary function of the body that is attempting to keep the penis healthy.

If these erections do not occur at all or in low number, or of poor rigid quality, this suggests an erectile dysfunction (ED) problem. If normal sleep erections occur, but a man is unable to become erect while awake, it usually indicates that the ED is due to a psychological cause. Men who have a physical cause (organic) for their ED will usually have some abnormality of the frequency, intensity, or duration of their erections while asleep.

So, we learn that erections are taking place during the night – perhaps up to six times a night – and our clothing and sleep posture can influence these erection that occur about every 90 minutes. Anything that you do, or not do, that can prevent pressure, restriction, or inability for the erect penis to fully straighten out, will be of immense and frequent benefit to your PD.

With this in mind, here are two new rules for you to follow:

1. Do not sleep face down. Sleeping on your tummy is bad for two primary reasons:

    A. Your neck must be sharply twisted to the side for hours at a time, when you sleep face down. This can lead to neck and shoulder problems.

    B. Your penis will get jammed and pressed against the mattress. Your erection has no where to go and, because you are in deep REM sleep, you are less likely to wake up and roll over to correct this problem.

2. Wear loose clothing, or no clothing, while you sleep.

    A. Wear just loose pajama bottoms, with no underwear.

    B. Wear nothing – sleep like you were born – naked.

    C. Wear loose underwear – no "Tightie Whities" or jockey-style underwear. Wear only loose boxer shorts; even these can cause some binding and restriction problems. It just might be best to follow B., above.

Getting "It" In and Out of Your Pants

Can you believe it? You are now actually going to read in some detail how to get your penis in and out of your pants. Sure, you have done it maybe 78,483 times in your life. And now you are going to read instructions for something that you do so well, you do not even have to think about it. Is this really necessary? Yep, because you are probably doing it incorrectly, since you have special needs because of your PD. If you did not have PD, perhaps it would not make much difference. However, so many things in a man's life change with PD, even getting ready to take a "leak."

This is perhaps the strangest, most personal and most labored instruction in this book. There was debate before writing this section about the depth of discussion to use, since it should be sufficient to state, "Be more careful when preparing to urinate," and not go into any details. For many men, however, that warning or explanation would have actually meant absolutely nothing. Some people are not mechanically inclined or creative enough to understand exactly what "being careful" means. Other people, for a variety of reasons, simply need greater detail and instruction. Some might think this is a discussion with a lot more detail than it deserves. Some would say it is not even necessary to discuss this topic since there is only one way to remove the penis from behind the clothing – you know, you just "do it." However, that would be a shortsighted assumption.

How you remove and return your penis through that small and irregular opening, guarded all around by sharp metal teeth, in and out, in and out, many times a day, is probably the single most real threat to your penis you experience. Sexual intercourse might be a more forceful threat to the welfare of a penis that harbors a PD scar, but it is not done as frequently or as haphazardly as is the simple act of preparing to urinate.

You Must Change How You Do It

Initially, you might not think it is necessary to change how you urinate. But all you have to do is merely <u>think</u> about it seriously for a short while and the importance of this common act to your PD becomes obvious. Only you know what and how you are doing, and if you need to change your procedure. It is important to your eventual recovery that you are not stressing and injuring the very tissue you are trying to heal.

Remember that odd number that I placed at the start of this section, "78, 483" as the number of times that you might have had to remove yourself from your pants? Seems like a big number, right? Well, it is probably way too low! If you urinate six times a day while you are wearing pants, and you are 60 years old, you have actually performed this fast little penis extraction process about <u>131,400 times</u>! The number is much higher if you include the countless times you do the very same thing while wearing only underwear or only pajamas in the middle of the night.

That can be a lot of collective abuse if you are doing it roughly or incorrectly. You know a flag eventually wears out if it is left to flap in the wind for too long. What about the way you "whip out" your penis? Could this be one of the ways you have contributed to the injury of your penis? No one will know for sure. Yet, if you are really interested in getting over your PD, why on earth would you take a chance and continue to abuse your scarred and bent penis every time you urinate?

Let's get down to the basics with a few questions:

1. Who taught you how to get your penis out of your pants? (Didn't I warn you that this discussion would be very basic and intimate?)

2. How do you actually get your penis out of your pants? What are the exact steps you usually follow to get the job done?

3. Do you have one technique for when you are flaccid or non-erect?

4. Do you have another technique for when you have an erection?

5. Do you have a technique for when you are in a real hurry and must rush to go to the bathroom?

6. Do you have yet another technique for when your pants are really tight or you are really tangled up in there?

An interesting subject when you think about it, isn't it? Let us go down the list and consider these topics in the order of the questions.

Who Taught You How to Get Your Penis Out of Your Pants?

I guarantee this answer will provide some insight into how you have been doing this little trick all of your life, and probably injuring yourself each time you do it.

So, again, who actually taught you how to slip your penis in and out of your pants when you must urinate? Probably no one actually showed you. Sure your mother probably was standing over you and telling you to pee in the potty, but do you really think she said, "Now, Junior, this is how you should pull your little penis out of your underwear. You must be careful, lest you develop Peyronie's disease. No, no, Sweetie, don't 'hook it' with your fingers and pull it through. Make some room and gently bring your precious little cargo out into the light. Make sure the opening of your pants is very wide, do not bend or pull too hard, and…"

No, she didn't say anything like that – of course not. She was rushed for time, and aggravated that you were probably peeing on the floor. Your Mom at this point in her life was tired of the whole potty training routine, and just wanted to make supper. She never said a word about how to <u>actually handle your penis</u>. After all, how could she know, she didn't own one.

<u>You were the one who figured it out for yourself</u>. It was just something you did as a very young boy of 2-3 years or so. You did it in a hurried, direct, aggressive, clumsy, and awkward way as any child would naturally do it.

How you started doing this simple and frequent process as a child is probably exactly how you continue to do it today. Why should it be any other way? At what point in your life would you otherwise stop and evaluate this process and decide to change your ways, were it not for having PD or reading a book such as this one? You are 67 years old and you are still peeing like you did when you were three years old. Amazing when you think about it, isn't it?

What a thought. You probably slip your penis out of and into your pants today just like you did when you were three years old. Here you are a successful lawyer, a bank president, a respected teacher, and you do this simple thing very much the same way you have always done it from early childhood. Not really classy, not very carefully, not very gently, but probably very direct and fast. This description makes sense to anyone who has been around a three year old boy – rough, tough, direct, don't slow me down because I have important things to do and urinating is not one of them.

So that should put things in perspective. You are probably yanking and pulling and stretching yourself like a kid. No wonder you have PD. You have to stop that, right now. Consider that an order from your mother.

Exact Steps to Get Your Penis Out of and into Your Pants

Every man knows about the unstated but strong cultural and survival prohibitions while standing at a urinal. You do not talk to strangers; maybe you can talk to someone you know who is with you, but probably not too much. You look straight ahead at the wall, and you do not make eye contact. You walk right up, open the zipper, dig in for your apparatus, do your business, you give it three shakes maximum, and then you walk away. Oh, yes, don't forget to wash your hands. While you are in the public restroom, to get caught observing another man's private parts is frowned upon and potentially risky.

In writing this book I have had to learn a few generalizations that probably cover the vast majority of techniques and attitudes about the private techniques men use to urinate. Bear in mind that I have had to be most careful and discreet in this research. Most of it is done out of the extreme corner of one eye, while keeping the head pointed straight, but the eyes straining hard to the right or left. There are limitations of observation, and very limited conversation – as you can well imagine. I have not felt brave enough to ask a stranger in a public restroom how he actually goes about extracting his penis from his pants.

It is safe to assume that the technique that anyone uses is the same if he is at home in total privacy or in a large 12 urinal public restroom. Here is the limited information I have learned:

1. Unzipping the pants is a one- or two-handed procedure.

2. The actual removal of the penis from the pants is most often a one-handed procedure.

3. Not much time or effort is spent in opening the pants fully, once the zipper is down. Probably the zipper is only partially opened.

4. Often a man will do a fancy little dance step while reaching into his pants for his penis. The little dance is a pretty standard event for those who do it. It goes like this:

   A. Quickly bend either knee just a little. At the same time rotate that leg outward a little, so the crotch area is very slightly and briefly flared opened.

   B. The knee that is bent and then rotated outward will be on the same side as the hand that is used to reach in for the penis.

   C. While the hand is reaching in for the penis, the low back is arched slightly and the buttocks are stuck out to make more room for the hand that is intruding into this tight area.

5. Most men seem to hold their penis while urinating.

   A. One-hand technique – seems to be a fast combination movement to unzip, reach in and grab penis

   B. Two-hand technique – while one hand unzips the other opens the "fly" or opening of the pants a little more, then the hand that was used to unzip continues to reach in to withdraw the penis.

6. The few men who do not hold their penis while urinating seem to put one hand on their hip, and they also look around a little.

7. Most men do not look down at their own penis while urinating. If a man looks down while he is urinating it is a very brief peek.

8. About 50% of men will stand with their legs spread considerably farther apart than when they stand while not urinating.

9. Returning the penis to the pants is also a very fast process. More time is spent zipping the zipper than getting the penis back into the pants.

   A. One-hand technique – seems to be a fast combination movement to open the "fly" with the back of the hand while the fingers push laterally to replace the penis to its congested resting area.

   B. Two-hand technique – while one hand opens the "fly" or opening of the pants a little more, the hand guides it back.

10. Returning the penis to the pants is usually accompanied by another fancy little dance step that has more to do with the pelvis. While the one- or two-hand technique is being done, the low back is arched, buttocks are stuck out, and both knees are bent slightly and quickly. This serves to allow more space for the return of the penis. It is almost as though the pelvis and penis are brought back together, while the zipper is kept in place so that the penis is drawn back in without touching it.

11. It appears that when the penis is not placed back into the pants with the hand, or guided through the tight opening of the clothes, it is actually pulled back into place by the movement of the pelvis that pushed back in the dance described in 10., above. In this technique, it appears that the penis almost goes back into the pants by itself.

Now that you have been presented with some description of how this common activity is performed, it will be interesting for you to slow down the next time you are in front of a toilet or urinal and dissect the steps that you actually use. See what you can and should do differently. Caution and care are the by-words.

Dangerous Undercover Work

Propriety and fear of being attacked have prevented further investigation of actual finger techniques and ways of touching the penis while it is in the pants.

What is most apparent in this whole process is that the entire act of urinating is performed in a rapid, rough and mechanical manner without much apparent attention being paid to what is being done. It seems to be a very hazardous time for the penis.

While sexual activity might certainly involve more forceful trauma, it occurs less often and appears to be less stressful to the penis since the anatomical relationships and lubrication tend to minimize injury. The manner that the penis is moved out and in around the tight corners and recesses of the cloth enclosures causes it to be pulled and stretched around several tight angles and corners each time a man urinates. Rough stuff.

You would think not much variation or personal style is used to get in and out of a car, or in and out of the shower, or in and out of a coat. Yet if you watch closely as people do these simple common activities, you will see many small but significant variations. Probably some things a person does to get into the shower or into a shirt were initially conscious decisions based on speed, comfort, convenience, body type, fluidity of movement, or whatever, at an early point in life, but now are done automatically. Later in life no thought or careful consideration is given to how any of these things are done – until, of course, a problem arises when a shoulder gets sore or a cast is on a hand and the usual way of doing something no longer is possible or makes sense.

Any new way of doing an old procedure is a difficult compromise to learn. However, it should be seen as a necessary improvement, and a solution for the problem that prompted the change. Eventually these new methods become as speedy, comfortable, and automatic as the old techniques they replaced.

How about your own particular personal method of getting your penis in and out of your pants when you stand to urinate? By now you know that you should slow down and be more careful. So let's consider a few things that you could be doing better for yourself.

Think about these small individual steps that should be improved as you remove your "cargo" from the tight spot it sits in all day long.

1. Slow down. Do not be so much in a rush that you injure yourself further.

2. Take your time to unzip your pants so the opening is as full as possible. Then open the fly as much as you can.

3. Use two hands. Open the pants and underwear openings wider than you usually do, using both hands. Use one to fully open the "fly" of your pants and underwear, as well as reposition the bottom end of your shirt that sometimes gets in the way, and the other hand to carefully extract your penis from your pants with several fingers, not just a one-fingered hook, in such a way that no stretching, tugging or twisting takes place.

4. Do not use just one finger to "hook around" your penis to pull it through the opening of your underwear and pants.

5. Slowly and carefully navigate your penis out so that it does not have to be stretched or traumatized every time you urinate.

6. Do not force your penis through the small opening of your underwear and pants by stretching it around tight folds of clothing that block its easy exit.

7. If you find that you are twisted, or folded around someway so that you cannot easily extract yourself, take the time to gently probe and examine how to remove yourself. Spend an extra five seconds to protect yourself.

This should be a new way of approaching an old and familiar routine. It is part of your job, to do what is necessary to get well. Will this cure your PD? No, probably not. But you can easily see this simple change of routine will prevent you from re-injuring yourself several times a day.

These suggestions and options are not perfect, nor are they complete. It is not known how the average man does these things. How you do your own personal extraction is known only to you, and it is you who must decide how to manage this process carefully.

These suggestions are presented to prevent mistakes that can easily worsen your PD or reverse any recovery you are trying to make with your problem. They are offered because the usual methods that most men resort to are not good for the PD sufferer, since they seldom consider the damaging consequences of frequent pulling, stretching, and tugging on the penis.

The Art of Urinating When You Have PD

When speaking to men who have PD, many times they admit they push, pull, and unbend the penis to straighten themselves out to urinate. No explanation is offered as to why they do this, and no questions are asked about purpose or motivation. Most of the time I assume this forceful unbending is a response to dissatisfaction and dread with the misshapen appearance of the penis at that time.

As we sometimes discuss these issues of forceful unbending, these men are surprised to learn this could be harmful. Thus we present some very fundamental instructions about a very fundamental function of life.

This section is presented last for a reason. Some of what is covered next can be considered gross and unusual. The reader by now should understand the intent is instruction and education to protect an injured body part, not an exercise in weird activities.

Each technique suggested is a compromise or tactic with the higher goal of reducing the potential for additional injury. If you understand the reason behind these novel ideas, they become less strange and more easily adopted.

First, About the Person You Live with

When PD enters into a relationship, interpersonal tension and marital stress are not always due to sexual problems alone. Family discord and interpersonal stress develop from a wide range of problems that intensify and accumulate because PD intensifies many other problems related and unrelated to PD. Marriages are wracked and ruined by fits of anger and violence, moodiness and shame so deep that all communication stops, intensification of unrelated problems that were present before the PD started, and (surprise!) personal hygiene problems.

If a man has low standards of personal hygiene and he is not considerate of his mate, this would probably extend itself into the bathroom. Urinating on the floor and toilet seat without cleaning up afterward can certainly place unreasonable stress on family members who must endure yet one more hardship and inconvenience because of his PD.

Women frequently complain about men not throwing their socks in the hamper after being told countless times to do so. It must be something that we all do instinctively. If you are guilty of such an inconsideration then you need to take stock of yourself and your attitude.

Your mate has to go through this terrible disease process with you. She must also endure stressful changes in her life and limitations of sexual contact, just as you are. There is no reason to add to her distress and burden by acting like an untrained puppy that pees all over the bathroom and then leaves it for her to deal with.

Big and small stresses accumulate in a marriage that is being tested by the addition of PD. Urine on the floor or toilet seat does not have to be one of them. Grow up and be a man. Be scrupulously clean about yourself. You owe it to her. It is the least you can do.

The stress of PD on both partners in a relationship can be enormous. A man who is not considerate of others in the bathroom creates a totally avoidable problem, even when he is already feeling so very guilty and ashamed of a problem he cannot avoid. Small acts of disrespect and inconsideration accumulate rapidly until just one more dirty toilet seat becomes the final straw that breaks her spirit.

If you want your wife to stand with you during this ordeal, you need to be considerate and respectful of her. PD is a big enough burden, do not create more.

"Water, Water Everywhere, but Not a Drop to Drink"

First, we need to consider the actual fluid that passes from your body, urine. Urine is commonly thought of as "dirty," a waste product, not to be touched. Remember how your mother made sure that you washed your hands after you used the restroom? "Don't touch anything" in the public restroom, remember? It left a strong message that everything in there was bad, and urine became a part of that impression.

But, in truth, urine is not dirty. It is cleaner, in many ways, than the water that you often drink in restaurants, with fewer bacteria and no foreign matter. In cases of kidney or urinary infection the urine will contain one or more kinds of bacteria, but otherwise urine as it leaves the body is virtually sterile and nearly odorless. This is why solders are instructed to cleanse their own wounds in battle with a stream of urine, since it is nearly sterile. In the traditional style of medicine practiced in India it is sometimes recommended for an ill person drink a small amount of his or her own fresh urine, a practice called "amaroli." It has been done for thousands of years, and is most acceptable in Indian culture.

It is only after the urine leaves you body and is allowed to sit for a while, that the bacteria of the outside environment contaminate the urine. Then, once outside the body, these bacteria convert naturally occurring chemicals in the urine into foul-smelling chemicals that we usually associate with stale urine. In particular, it is the ammonia in stale urine that has the offensive odor. Ammonia comes from odorless urea that is produced from protein in the body.

We need to keep in mind that much of our repulsion about urine is from strong cultural messages and misconceptions, and not the reality of it.

So when you are dealing with different ways of urinating and necessary compromises, you are not dealing with a toxic substance. If you wash your hands and practice good hygiene after you urinate, you are not doing anything abnormal or dirty.

Urination Is Complicated by Changes in the Penis

PD rarely causes a curve or bend in the penis while non-erect, or flaccid; any curvature present in the flaccid state is typically minor. These small deviations are usually not a problem during urination since the penis is soft and pliable. The penis can be turned easily to direct the urine stream in the appropriate direction.

The most common direction for the penile distortion during erection is for it to turn upward, since most scars are on the top of the shaft. Many curve to the left, right, or downward, but the most frequent distortion reported is toward the ceiling. Additionally, the curve can be a compound curvature, meaning it can be distorted in two different planes at the same time. In PD, a penis can bend to the left and up, or to the right and down, or any of several combinations. Further, these penile distortions can extend into a considerable degree of curvature. At the extreme, men have such severe curvature during erection the pattern is referred to as a "cane handle distortion." The distortion patterns can be variable and extreme from case to case, as well as variable from time to time even in the same individual.

These various distortions present a challenge during urination because they do not often send the stream in a straight forward pattern, but in the direction of penile deviation projecting to the left, right, and most often upward toward the ceiling.

Thus, a man with PD has his greatest problem urinating while he has an erection. Complicating this situation, during erection not much can be done to alter the deviated course of urine flow because the penis is rigid. When erect it is not easy to make much correction in the curvature, and it is not a good thing to do anyway. The erect bent penis should never be unbent or changed in anyway at anytime, least of all in a case of PD.

<u>Never attempt to push, unbend or change the position of the erect penis in an effort to redirect the urine stream</u>. The reason is the thin but tough tissue membrane inside the penis (known as the tunica albuginea, the actual layer that becomes injured and develops the PD scar) is most vulnerable while it is stretched tightly during an erection.

Think of it this way: Is a balloon more likely to be punctured if it is under-inflated or over-inflated? Sure, it can be damaged easier when it is stretched out tightly. Although the actual mechanism of injury is not a puncture of the penis, the principle of vulnerability is the same. The tunica albuginea is made of multiple laminated layers. At the points where the different sections of the tunica come in contact with each other, these layers can become separated or "delaminated." This is how the whole PD problem often starts.

Therefore, never try to push the erect penis up, down to the sides or straighten the bend, because you can stress this tight membrane in the penis. This is not the time or technique to help the situation, or help yourself. Better ways of controlling and directing the urine stream exist; we will get into these shortly.

Urinating with a Crooked Erection

If you have PD and do not understand the need for this particular discussion, consider yourself lucky. Many men with severe PD distortion (cane-handle or corkscrew deformity) experience such a problem while urinating they cannot easily manage the stream relative to the orientation or position of their body.

Men are notorious for peeing on toilet seats anyway, but the chances are so much greater when the penis is crooked. Relax: this is not the beginning of a lecture about lifting the toilet seat. Getting the toilet seat out of the way might help the toilet seat issue, but with PD the additional problem of pee on the floor, walls, clothes, shoes, and other places can occur. There appears to be two problems with urination in PD and both are much greater than a faulty aim. The problem is the barrel of the gun is bent and shoots consistently off target compared to your prior lifelong experience, and the second is that many men sometimes do not clean up after themselves.

For a man with a crooked penis to urinate, the most direct and stubborn strategy to temporarily manage this problem is by forcibly correcting the curvature to about where it should be and then begin urinating. For any logically-minded man this would be a good way of handling the problem. However, it is an extremely bad decision and a very good way to cause more problems for the penis. It might be logical and it might make a man feel for a moment that things are back to normal, but he runs a huge risk of making his problem worse.

The guiding principle is very simple: <u>When urinating with a distorted penis, change anything else you need to change, but do not attempt to change the penis</u>.

Below are specific ideas for addressing the matter of urinating with a bent erection. Some are rather obvious, some rather unusual, one or two might not appeal to you, but they will prevent you from peeing all over the bathroom. They have been listed in the order of simplicity and ease of using these suggestions:

1. Perhaps the easiest solution is to wait a minute or two to see if the erection will subside before urinating. A non-erect penis is easier to deal with than an erect penis.

2. Slow down. Do not be so much in a rush that you injure yourself further.

3. Avoid using a public urinal. When using a public urinal a man will be given less opportunity to adapt to his personal needs without looking and feeling peculiar. You are more inclined to feel like you want to bend your penis if you are standing at a public urinal, rather than simply standing off-center or turned away from the urinal while urinating into it.

4. Use an enclosed private toilet where you can address personal issues without being observed. Within the privacy of the enclosed space you are less inclined to have an accident while urinating and you can tend to yourself in whatever way is necessary.

5. Stand off-center, or rotate at an angle to the toilet so the stream of urine will be compensated for correctly. If your curve is to the left, stand to the right or turn your body to the right to position your steam to hit your target, and of course, the opposite if you are curved of the right.

6. Sit while urinating, especially with an erection that bends down.

7. Take the time to unzip your pants all the way so the opening is as full as possible. Then open the fly as much as you can.

8. Use two hands to extract the penis. Open the pants and underwear wide, using both hands. Use one to fully open the "fly" of your pants and underwear, as well as reposition the bottom end of your shirt that sometimes gets in the way. With the other hand carefully remove your penis from your pants.

9. If your penile curvature is so bad that urinating is a messy or problematic, use small inexpensive plastic bags in a few effective ways:

   A. Place only the head of the penis inside the bag, holding the bag closed around the head of the penis so urine will go directly into the bag. The surrounding area will say clean and dry.

   B. Place the bag over your hand like glove or puppet and hold the palm of your hand over the opening of the penis (almost like you hold Kleenex tissue over your nose when you are going to blow your nose) and then urinate so the urine hits the bag, immediately falling into the toilet. You are basically deflecting the urine against your hand in such a way that it can only go down. NOTE: Do not flush the plastic bag down the toilet.

10. If you have the convenience of using equipment at home, several options are available that make it easier to urinate:

A. Urinate into a large bucket or container that can be emptied into the toilet, washed, rinsed and put away until the next use.

B. Urinate against a curved surface – a sheet of plastic, a small bowl, or a cup – and angle that surface you are urinating against so that the urine is deflected down into the toilet.

C. Urinate into a hand-held portable male urinal that has a wide opening and a deep reservoir; it can be washed, rinsed and put away until the next use; you can buy one at any drug store for just a few dollars.

11. If you have to urinate away from home, without the convenience of using your equipment, other options are available:

A. If you know you are going to be away from home, prepare for when you will have to urinate; bring supplies:

1) A plastic bag – to pee in and then dump or to put over your hand like a glove to urinate against, and deflect down into the toilet.

3) Disposable handy-wipe paper towels that come wrapped in a sealed pouch to clean yourself up.

4) Urinate into a large wad of toilet paper that is placed over the head of the penis and held over the toilet so the urine will fall into the toilet.

5) Urinate against your own hand and angle the palm so the urine is deflected down into the toilet. Is this gross and offensive? Perhaps, but remember that urine is practically sterile and has no special odor most of the time. Tactics such as this are smarter than urinating on your pants or the floor, and it is far better than injuring yourself. Just like Mom told you so many times, do not forget to wash your hands.

12. When you urinate at home, here is an unorthodox and direct technique:

A. Urinate directly into the shower or bathtub.

B. Explain to your wife ahead of time what you are doing – how this is an easier and more desirable solution based on your needs, and then do it.

C. Stand at the very edge of your shower or bathtub, arch your back and stick your pelvis out as much possible so that your penis is well over and into the enclosed space of the shower or bathtub.

D. When you are sure you will not make a mistake, urinate right in the shower stall or bath tub. Be careful to evaluate the splashing of urine. Find an angle at which you can direct your stream so that the urine stays contained within that space and does not splash outside to cause odor problems later.

E. Afterward, run water to wash the urine away thoroughly.

F. Let your partner know what you did and that you cleaned up after yourself. She will appreciate your consideration for taking these extra steps to make sure you and the bathroom stays clean.

You must decide how important it is to get over your PD and what you are willing to do to manage this problem in a direct and positive manner. Once you have decided, as I did, that getting over this lousy problem is the most important goal in your life, then all of the other decisions are easy. Anything and everything makes sense if it is directed toward overcoming PD, even if it would be something you would never do before.

What about the young fellow who was in a mountain climbing accident, trapped between rocks for days, and amputated his own leg? Once he realized he had only two choices to make – self-amputation or death – he said it became very clear what he had to do, and he simply did it.

You do what you have to do.

Chapter 7 – Take Vitamins for PD Like This…

Ω **- To live a better life, be happier and healthier in spite of your PD, and increase your chance of successfully treating it …**

… you should support your health and ability to heal and repair in as many ways as you possibly can. One of the most important aspects of increasing your ability to heal – your immune capability – is to improve your nutritional intake every day. "You are what you eat" not only makes a lot of sense, but science agrees with this idea. Our study indicates that many men with PD have a history of poor digestion. Go to the **PDI** *web site for a complete description of all that you should consider doing for yourself nutritionally. This chapter gives you the basic information about what supplements you can take, how to take them, and what to watch out for, while you are improving your nutritional intake.*

Talk to Your Doctor

First and foremost, it is most important for you to inform your doctor of all aspects of the nutritional treatment plan you are undergoing. **PDI** cannot be your doctor, and this book cannot and does not make specific details for your care. Only you and your family physician or urologist can take responsibility for your eventual treatment. This section consists of suggestions, ideas and general health topics that should be given final approval by your doctor before you make any changes to your therapy program.

At no time should you tolerate feeling nauseated or uncomfortable with abdominal distress or diarrhea because you are treating your PD with Alternative Medicine therapies. If you experience nausea, diarrhea, gas, bloating, or similar symptoms that you suspect are being caused by the nutritional products you are taking, it indicates the possibility of some level of irritation or dysfunction occurring in your digestive system. If your GI tract is irritated and dumping out its contents as fast as you put it in, you cannot possibly absorb the good nutrients you are consuming. You must make sure that your digestive system feels good, and functions well, so it is able to absorb all of the nutrients you are taking.

Your effort should be directed not only to taking care of yourself so that you feel good, but you should also consider that you can only fully take advantage of your PD therapy program if your digestive system is functioning well to absorb these special nutrients.

Taking a Lot of Pills

The problem of abdominal distress (nausea, bloating, diarrhea, gas) occurs for certain sensitive individuals, because of taking the aggressive dosages of multiple supplements that are necessary to gain the desired therapeutic benefit. A higher dosage is often used because taking a lower dosage usually does not achieve the desired results with PD.

Abdominal distress also arises because it is often necessary in Alternative Medicine to take several courses of different therapies at the same time, which are often unique to the diet (Chinese herbs). The body must get used to the higher levels of these nutritional and enzyme supplements, and substances that are foreign to the diet. Also, this type of Alternative Medicine therapy can bring on side-effects related to pushing toxins out of the tissue. Hence, this information will guide you through this process.

Most PD treatment plans that are described on the **PDI** web site using enzymes and nutritional supplements are aggressive and are used frequently with and between meals throughout the day. Occasionally, for some men with a tendency toward digestive complaints, or those who have high metabolic tissue toxicity, this level of intense enzyme and nutritional supplementation can cause temporary and mild side-effects: diarrhea, gas, abdominal pain, or other similar symptoms are the most commonly reported problems. More often, it is our experience that if such a response is related to detoxification then other secondary symptoms can also occur in the early stages of a PD treatment plan as the result of release of tissue toxins into the general circulation: mild itching and/or rash, bad breath, or so much greater energy that sleep is sometimes difficult.

If you should experience any of the above listed symptoms, or any unusual reaction that cannot be otherwise explained, **PDI** strongly advises that you temporarily stop taking the product you suspect might be causing the problem. Completely stop taking that product and wait for the problem to not only improve, but to completely cease. You want the problem/symptom to completely disappear for at least 48 hours before you even begin to think about taking any more of the same product that is suspected to be causing the side effect to flare up. If after you stop taking the product for 48 hours, and the problem continues to worsen to any degree, call your family doctor. When you stop taking the product, the problem/symptoms should begin to calm down in 24-48 hours. Again, to avoid misunderstanding or confusion: within 24-48 hours of stopping the product, the problem/symptom should at least begin to improve, even if it is not gone by then; improvement should start within a day or two, even if it just continues to slowly improve from that point; if it starts improving then that is a good sign and you will then know that things are under control.

Relief from these reactions depends on your individual constitution and body chemistry. If it doesn't happen the way that is suggested – or if you start getting some other strong or strange reactions during the 24-48 hours after you stopped taking the supplements, like increase of heart rate or pounding headaches or blurry vision or lightheadedness – you must call your family doctor immediately.

Most Common Cause of a "Reaction"

It is most common for a reaction problem/symptom to begin simply because a person begins taking too much of a product initially, based on individual tolerance. Perhaps someone else can take a particular dose with no reaction, but another person finds that same dose to be excessive for him.

Continue to avoid the product you suspect is causing the problem/symptom for two whole days <u>after</u> your problem/symptom is gone. This does not mean you stop taking the product for two whole days; it means after the symptom/problem stops, then you start counting two more days on top of that to be sure your body is clear of that product and has a chance to recuperate. After feeling good, with no symptoms, for two whole days then consider taking ONE of that same product per day for 2-3 days. That's all, just one a day – no more. You should slowly and safely test the situation to determine how your body will respond to a very small dose. If you get a return of the problem/symptom at this very low dose, stop it again and stay off that product for a week. Then one week later try again at the same one per day dose. If you get a return of that same problem/symptom again, do not go back on it at all since it is likely something that you obviously have a sensitivity and cannot tolerate. However, this is all extremely rare.

The usual situation that we encounter involves a brief and mild initial reaction of diarrhea that is controlled by merely lowering the dose by one or two pills per day, just one step below the level of supplementation that the person was taking when the problem began. After this is done there is usually no problem returning to the dosage that caused the initial reaction, and even higher than that.

The great majority of men can take as much of a product as they need, if they just build up to it slowly and gradually.

Increasing Dosage over Time

If you wish to continue increasing the dose of a product that has caused some trouble in the past, then consider using this suggested guideline for re-introducing it into your plan.

If you experience no new problem and no return of the problem/symptom after taking just one a day for 2-3 days, then increase your dose slightly. Take just ONE product in the AM and ONE in the PM for 4-5 days. You are now taking <u>two</u> pills per day.

If you experience no return of the problem/symptom after taking this slightly increase in taking the product, then increase the dosage slightly. Then take ONE in the AM, ONE in mid-PM and ONE in late PM for 4-5 days. You are not taking <u>three</u> pills per day.

If you experience no return of the problem/symptom after taking this slightly increased dose of the product, then increase the dosage again slightly. Then take TWO in the AM and ONE in mid-PM and ONE in late-PM for 7-10 days. You are now taking <u>four</u> pills per day.

If you experience no return of the problem/symptom after taking this slightly increased dose of the product, then increase the dosage again slightly. Then take TWO in AM and TWO in mid-PM and ONE in late PM for 7-10 days. You are now taking <u>five</u> pills a day.

If you experience no return of the problem/symptom after taking this slightly increased dose of the product, then increase the dosage again slightly. Then take TWO in AM and TWO in mid-PM and TWO in late PM for 7-10 days. You are now taking six pills a day.

Can you see how this suggested strategy slowly and carefully works the dose up a little at a time?

At this point evaluate how far you wish to proceed with this process. You might want to think about increasing your dose to any higher level only if you have a strong reason to do so, and if your doctor approves.

If at any time you get a return of the problem/symptom while you are slowly increasing your dosage, then simply stop taking the product for 48 hours, and start from the beginning at the dose of one per day for a few days. But when you get to the highest dosage at which you were not getting the problem/symptom, go no further with the increase for maybe a few weeks. (In other words, get back up to the same dose when you were having no problems, and just stay there for a while). After 2-3 weeks at that dose, if you continue to feel good, then slowly try increasing the dosage again. You want to be SLOW AND CAREFUL with any of these products; they are all powerful in their own way.

The enzyme group especially works very well and can improve your physiology by simply increasing your circulation. You will never definitely know that any problem/symptom response that occurred was actually related to any particular product, but you want to be careful and safe. Your new symptom or suspected side-effect could have been perhaps just a coincidence, or caused by something else that you did or ate, or something that would have happened to you no matter what you were doing at the time. You will never really know for sure. But, better safe than sorry. Using the very safe and conservative approach you will give your body time to adjust and adapt to the increased blood circulation and the detoxification that may be occurring as a result of your treatment plan.

Do not feel urgency to reach any particular dose of these Alternative Medicine therapies; there is no magic dose of any product. If it happens that the most of any product you can take in a day is just 1 or 2 capsules, and that particular dose is making your circulation better or your PD is better in some other way, then what difference does the number of pills make? The important thing is that you are feeling better and that you are doing so with a safe program of wellness. You want to methodically and slowly work your way back up to a safe and effective dose, with no problems or compromise to your health.

In the case where you can comfortably tolerate a particular product only at a relatively low dose, then you must accept that as "your" dose and not attempt to push to higher levels than what has been shown to be tolerable. No greater nutritional value comes from a dose higher than you are comfortable with, since it is not likely that you will absorb much of the product that you take at the higher level when you have diarrhea, gas and pain. You need to understand and accept the wisdom of your body, to listen to your body when it speaks to you, and be in harmony with it.

Work Problems

As a small and unrelated topic, another aspect of supplement dosage needs to be briefly covered at this point. This concerns the inability to closely follow your PD therapy plan because of work-related problems. Many men are pressed for time during the course of their work day, and can't stop at work to take their supplements. Others are unable to keep all the different supplements in their plan nearby. They have great difficulty following their plan because of these restrictions.

To solve some of these problems men have tried to take all, or most, of their supplements at one time. This can be a big mistake. Good therapy plans for PD are large, involving a variety of different supplements, especially the systemic enzymes. The digestive tract often cannot tolerate taking a massive dose of these. How many therapy products a person can take is dictated by the ability of the digestive tract to absorb and assimilate these products at one time. Merely loading the digestive system out of convenience is not a good strategy. Usually, shall we say, it backfires in a bad case of diarrhea due to the overload. This causes a lot of other work-related problems.

It is not easy for some men to treat their PD with frequent supplementation, self-administered acupuncture treatment, DMSO and hot packs, the way they would like to do it. With work and time restrictions it is sometimes impossible to solve all problems and restrictions of someone's employment. Using creativity and ingenuity, a compromise is often devised that attempts to keep as close as possible to the guidelines that we suggest for using these products. It all comes down to determination and how badly you want to solve your PD problem. As an example, it just might be necessary for a man to either get to bed earlier or get less sleep, in order to find the extra time to follow his PD therapy routine. For most people there comes a time and point where a decision is made that nothing is more important than confronting the problem, and then everything else falls easily into place.

Supplements on the Go

Often it is part of a good solution to take your supplements along with you to work in a shirt pocket, or kept with you where you work, in a small hard plastic carrying case. These are available on the **PDI** web site where all of the supplements are found. By taking one or two or even three of these cases with you when you leave the house at the beginning of the day, you can have your entire day planned out and ready for you.

Then it is merely a matter of remembering to stop and pop the pills at the appropriate time.

Taking Supplements All at Once or Spread out

To get the most out of your PD therapy plan, you must first understand that not all the "pills" in a PD therapy plan are in the same category; since these pills are in two different categories, (food and enzymes), they are taken differently. When you order your nutritional or "food" therapy and your enzyme therapy supplements from PDI, a sheet of complete written instructions is enclosed with your order to assure you know exactly how to take each product.

Food – One large category of "pills" is made up of general nutritional products that can be thought of as "food." These are the vitamins, minerals and related nutrients the body needs to constantly build and rebuild all tissues to stay healthy. Examples are vitamins E and C, PABA, and nutrients that are found in the food we eat. And just like food, these nutritional products should be taken with meals.

Some men think that if they have to take a total of six pills per day, it would be easier to just take them all at once. While this may be more convenient, it may cause trouble because there are limits to how much nutrition a body can absorb and assimilate at one time. It would be like sitting down in the morning to eat breakfast, lunch and dinner at the same time, so you would not have to stop to eat for the rest of the day. This sounds like a very efficient idea, but it is not reasonable. Instead, just like animals in the wild, we humans really should eat a little bit all day long, because it makes for better absorption of food. And so it is with the nutritional products we take for PD. It is usually a far better strategy to take the nutritional therapy products more often during the day, in evenly divided doses, so a portion of the supplements are taken with each meal. In this way the nutrients in the pills are incorporated with your food, for better absorption.

Six "food" pills, taken two at a time with meals throughout the day, are better than six pills taken all at one time. Most people will just divide their total nutritional therapy pills equally among the two or three meals they eat each day.

Enzymes – These also are "pills," but they are different from the nutrients that come in pill form. These enzyme "pills" are not nutrients in the way that vitamin E or copper are in the body. Enzymes in a PD therapy plan are taken for the sole purpose of removing the imperfectly formed foreign protein of the penile scar. The trick in taking these enzymes is to limit their contact with food in the digestive tract, since they would be used by the body to break down the proteins, fats and carbohydrates they contact. Any enzymes used in food digestion would not be available to help your PD. For this reason it is best to put these enzymes into your body, and into your bloodstream, when there is no food present in your digestive tract. When the enzymes have no where else to go, and nothing else to do other than enter the general blood system, they will remove imperfectly formed proteins like the PD scar. This is why we refer to these as "systemic enzymes"; they are to be used throughout all the systems and areas of your body, not just the digestive tract.

Since the enzymes of a PD plan are not intended to digest food, they are taken between meals. In fact, the idea is to carefully pay attention to the time of the last meal and the next meal, so they can be free to roam and circulate throughout your body systems, clearing up as many foreign proteins as possible. Usually, it is best to take these systemic enzymes one hour, or more, before you eat, and one hour, or more, after you eat.

However, there is another way of taking the systemic enzymes to increase their ability to remove the scar material, other than evenly distributing them between meals throughout the day. The exact method must be determined by each person through trial and error. This other method involves taking the systemic enzymes in larger groups, and less often – if your digestive tract can handle the presence of a large amount of enzymes working at one time. The intent of this strategy is to use a larger dose of systemic enzymes less frequently, than to use a smaller dose more frequently. It would be similar to the question, "What is the better way to clean my drain pipes? Should I flood the pipes with a large dose of drain cleaner once a month, or should I use a small amount of cleaner every week?" Both ideas have merit, but depending on circumstances one could work better than the other. What is the best way? Try both methods for a while and see which works better for you. That is what any scientist, or plumber, would tell you.

It may not always be practical, because a heavy dose of enzymes taken at once can be uncomfortable, but six "enzyme" pills, taken all at one time, might be better than taking one pill at six different times. Most people will experiment with the most comfortable dose they can manage during the end of the day; usually this is around half of the total they will take in any particular day. There are no magic doses of systemic enzymes to take; it is necessary for each person to determine what works best for him based on careful assessment and consultation with his treating doctor.

This is the reason for the special way of taking Neprinol® that is discussed on page 94 of this book.

If you are taking systemic enzymes, one or two at a time, between meals, and you do not detect progress with your PD, consider the possibility of experimenting with a larger group of them at a time between meals, but take them less often.

In other words, you can take a total of six Neprinol® in different patterns:

1. Two at a time between your three meals.

2. Two between breakfast and lunch, and later take four an hour or so before bedtime.

3. One between breakfast and lunch, one between lunch and dinner, and later take four an hour or so before bedtime.

In each pattern, the total is still six Neprinol®, but the strategy is much different – with perhaps different results. One might work better for you than the other. There is no way to know which will be more effective until you experiment a little.

Be sure to evaluate the patterns and timing of any supplements you take on the basis of your body's reaction to it. If you are nauseated, or develop diarrhea or abdominal pain after making a change in your therapy plan, then you must follow steps to reduce your discomfort by taking less of that supplement – probably just for a while until your body gets used to it. On the other hand, if you note favorable changes in the size, shape, density and contour of your scar after altering your plan in any way, then you must re-evaluate how to continue or even increase that part of your plan. Your body will let you know when you should make changes in your plan, based on the reactions of your body.

How will you know you are taking "pills" at the correct dose and at the correct time of day, in the most effective strategy? You closely monitor, judge, measure and watch your scar(s) to learn how it behaves while you gradually alter your therapy plan, looking for the pattern that caused your scar to change favorably. Return to page 33 for a review of how to monitor your PD scar, in order to know which pattern is effective for you. This is how you will know you have a truly effective and dynamic PD therapy plan. Go for it, my friend.

Schedule to Follow During the Day

Here are some basic rules and common sense information about taking any kind of multiple- or single-vitamin, mineral, systemic enzyme, amino acid, green drink or protein drink, or health food product in any kind of nutritional program.

Take these with meals (immediately before eating or during a meal):

1. Vitamins A, D, E, K, all the vitamins of the B group, vitamin C

2. Multiple vitamin supplements

3. Mineral and multiple mineral supplements, and specialty mineral products like MSM

4. Digestive enzymes and acid-containing preparations that you wish to assist your digestion of food

5. Bottom line: if you taking a nutritional product that comes from a food source (vitamin C from tomatoes, iron from meat) then eat it with food so that its absorption and assimilation can be increased

Take these between meals (1 hour or more before eating or 2 hours after eating):

1. Systemic enzymes that are taken to reduce foreign protein (plaque) or scars in the body

2. Homeopathic products which are meant to be taken when no food has recently been in the mouth, not even the taste or odor of food remains in the mouth.

3. Any product that bothers your digestion if you take it with food.

If you experience stomach distress, intestinal discomfort, diarrhea, or other unusual symptoms after taking any supplements, it is essential to determine which one(s) is the problem. Then take necessary steps to correct the problem, so you can continue taking all of the other supplements, after you determine you can do so safely.

The first step is to stop all the supplements you think are bothering you so that your digestive track settles down and behaves well for several days. After your digestive system has rested for a few days, then you need to test these same products to see what dose you can take without causing problems for yourself. Simply reintroduce the same products back into your therapy plan, but at a lower and slower rate of reintroduction.

At the start, consider taking a very low dose for a week or two. Slowly build the dose up over a period of a week or two at a time, and see what happens. If you are just very sensitive to a particular supplement, it might be necessary to stay permanently on a lower dose that does not upset your gut. This is usually a better strategy than just stopping it all together, because it is important you take in as much of this nutrient as you can. Better to take a little of a supplement so that it does not bother you (that you will likely absorb well because the digestive lining is not irritated), than take a lot of a supplement that bothers your digestive track (that you are not absorbing well any way because of the irritated digestive track).

From our experience two main problem areas occur with the supplements that can be used in a PD program:

1. Vitamin C – is an acidic supplement, ascorbic acid; some people cannot tolerate high levels of additional acid in the gut. If you develop diarrhea or other gastric distress, try lowering the dose of vitamin C to determine if this is helpful. If it does help you, then strongly consider taking the buffered vitamin C product **PDI** has available just for this reason. It is listed on the web site as "Ascorbplex 1000." This product change could make a significant difference to you.

2. Enzymes – taking these on an empty stomach can be too strong for some individuals. If you experience diarrhea or other gastric distress, try taking the enzymes closer to the time before or after eating so something is in your stomach to help absorb the enzyme activity.

Additional Considerations of the Therapy Plan During the Night

When I was most actively treating my PD, when my problem was at its worst and I was working the hardest to take in a very large number of therapy products during the day, I found two simple strategies to increase the effectiveness of the systemic enzyme segment of my therapy plan. These strategies make a lot of sense and are easy to incorporate.

1. **A different way of dividing enzymes during the day –**

    Let's say that you wish to take six Neprinol® systemic enzyme capsules in a day as your therapy dose. That is a good goal. Many men use that level and do well with it. Others do even better at nine or more a day of that product. For your general information, I have witnessed more success at the nine and above dose than at the six dosage level.

    If you wish to take six Neprinol® a day, and you know of course to take these between meals, you would logically take them in this way:

    > 2 Neprinol® – mid morning (between breakfast and lunch)
    > 2 Neprinol® – mid afternoon (between lunch and dinner)
    > + 2 Neprinol® – an hour or two after supper (or your last late night snack)
    > 6 Neprinol® total in a day

    This is good. But another system can be can be followed to take the same six Neprinol® per day that is probably more effective. Consider taking the same six Neprinol® in this way instead:

    > 1 Neprinol® – mid morning (between breakfast and lunch)
    > 2 Neprinol® – mid afternoon (between lunch and dinner)
    > + 3 Neprinol® – an hour or two after supper (or your last late night snack)
    > 6 Neprinol® total in a day

    The advantage of this pattern is that you are placing three Neprinol® in your system during a better time of day. You are creating a higher level of Neprinol® in your blood stream when you will have less food in your system, for a longer period of time, to be absorbed and work throughout your body. This way, it is more likely to get to the foreign fibrous protein material you would like it to attack. If you consider that after your last meal or snack of the day, you are without new additional food in your bloodstream for about 10-12 entire hours, this is a great time to load up on as much Neprinol® as you possibly can.

If you find that you can easily handle the three Neprinol® during the night (with no diarrhea) then consider this modification of the above plan:

> 1 Neprinol® – mid morning (between breakfast and lunch)
>
> 1 Neprinol® – mid afternoon (between lunch and dinner)
>
> + 4 Neprinol® – an hour or two after supper (or your last late night snack)
>
> 6 Neprinol® total in a day

Same number of total Neprinol® in a day, but perhaps better placement in your system when it can do the most for you. Not a bad strategy!

You can use any number of total Neprinol® during the day, with the same basic idea of taking fewer at a time during the day, and taking a higher number at the last dose of the day so you are most saturated during the long period of time during the night when your gut is empty the longest.

Here is how you would use a total of NINE Neprinol® in different patterns:

> 3 Neprinol® – mid morning (between breakfast and lunch)
>
> 3 Neprinol® – mid afternoon (between lunch and dinner)
>
> + 3 Neprinol® – an hour or two after supper (or your last late night snack)
>
> 9 Neprinol® total in a day

> 2 Neprinol® – mid morning (between breakfast and lunch)
>
> 3 Neprinol® – mid afternoon (between lunch and dinner)
>
> + 4 Neprinol® – an hour or two after supper (or your last late night snack)
>
> 9 Neprinol® total in a day

> 2 Neprinol® – mid morning (between breakfast and lunch)
>
> 2 Neprinol® – mid afternoon (between lunch and dinner)
>
> + 5 Neprinol® – an hour or two after supper (or your last late night snack)
>
> 9 Neprinol® total in a day

When I was taking heavy doses of Neprinol® when my problem was at its worst, and I had conditioned my digestive tract to handle these higher doses, I had no problem taking five Neprinol® at a time. Once that initial conditioning took place there was no number of Neprinol® that gave me a digestive problem.

2. Night time use of enzymes –

This is simply a suggestion that you can also take in an additional one or two Neprinol® or other nattokinase or serrapeptase product during the middle of the night when you are up to urinate anyway.

Bear in mind you must consider and adapt any additional nighttime Neprinol® with the dosage you take after the last meal of the day. Perhaps the additional one or two Neprinol® at 2-3AM will not be a problem if you took five Neprinol® at 8PM. Then again it might be more than you can tolerate. If you know you can handle it, great. Try it out and see what happens.

I found this did not cause any additional distress to my digestive system, and kept the level of systemic enzymes very high. I attribute a lot of my success over PD to this constant treatment approach, especially with the aggressive and continual use of Neprinol®.

Check with Your Doctor

We encourage you to talk to your personal physician about any digestive problem or concern you may have. It is critical that you keep your family doctor informed about your progress and your current condition, especially when you have a complicated medical history that presents a problem.

Lastly, please contact PDI via email if you have a question about your supplements. Do not telephone PDI; you will only be asked to submit your question in writing. We want to have a record not only of your question, we also need to document our communication with you. No information will be given about this or other problems over the phone, only in a written email format.

It is important to think long term, to stay with your program, and to be safe. Good luck with your treatment plan

Chapter 8 – Massage and Exercise for PD

Ω - **To live a better life, be happier and healthier in spite of your PD, and increase your chance of successfully treating it ...**

... you must do all that you can to increase your ability to heal and repair the tissue of the lower pelvis. Bringing in a good blood supply and assuring a good drainage of waste products from that area is vital to your general health and well-being, as well as your recovery effort. PDI has developed some fast, easy, simple ways for you to exercise and massage the tissue of the lower pelvis to assist your recovery from PD. This chapter gets you started on a most important part of the larger overall plan for your success in beating this terrible problem.

Two Common and Easy Therapies Apply

Two common and very simple therapies, that have been used for centuries for a wide variety of health problems, are never mentioned in the treatment of PD. These therapies increase the speed and extent of recovery in a wide variety of cases, from severe skin burns to emotional problems, yet are never discussed in the standard medical PD literature as potential therapies. These two overlooked therapies are massage and exercise. It just goes to show how traditional medicine is fixed only toward drugs and surgery as a cure for PD (and most all other health problems).

This chapter will correct this oversight. You will be instructed how to use massage and exercise in treatment of PD. Use this information to improve your pelvic muscle tone and circulation easily and effectively.

The broad appeal of massage and exercise comes from their ability to increase oxygen at the cellular level by improving the blood supply, and reduce toxin accumulation by improving drainage of venous blood and lymphatic fluid, as well as improve immune function by stimulation of endorphin production. Either, or both, are often applied to specific diseased or weakened areas of the body, such as in stroke cases or emphysema, and are used generally for the entire body when appropriate, such as in Parkinson's disease or Restless Leg Syndrome. Since the penis is composed of soft tissue and has a rich blood supply, it would certainly seem logical that both could be an appropriate treatment.

There are reasons for the absence of massage and exercise in PD treatment within the standard medical community, even though they are time-tested in many hundreds of health problems. Medical doctors in the U.S. tend to be all about medication and surgery, especially when it involves high-tech systems and wonder-drugs. Seldom are low-tech therapies given as much attention: they offer little financial incentive; they provide no excitement or glamour in applying simple therapies that have been used countless times for the treatment of other diseases; it takes effort and considerable time to explain massage and exercise techniques, especially those you will find in the next sections of this chapter; lastly, nothing is faster and easier for a doctor to do than write a simple prescription for another medication.

Deep Tissue Massage for PD

When I discuss deep tissue massage for PD with someone, one of the first questions is how hard the scar should be massaged. The natural assumption is that any massage to be effective in PD must be directly applied to the scar, perhaps like ironing the scar out of the penile tissue. Nothing could be further from the truth.

No massage or pressure is ever to be applied to the scar, or the penis, when using a massage technique in treatment of PD.

Two reasons dictate avoidance of direct contact to the penis. The first is that direct contact with the penis is not necessary, since it is the tissue in the surrounding areas of the lower pelvis that are of concern due to their often contracted and tense condition. The second reason is that it is not worth the risk to apply any type of repeated or extended pressure or force to the PD scar.

Since a man with a PD lesion in the penile tissue has already demonstrated he is capable of overreaction and scar development, it is not wise to do anything to provoke that same tissue with further potential injury. Most men with PD do not recall an injury or trauma that could have started their problem, not even a minor event. It is not uncommon to learn from someone with PD that his problem came soon after a medical procedure called catheterization, in which a probe device is passed up the urethra or urinary passage of the penis. This is a rather simple procedure that does not exert much force or stretching of the penile membranes, yet it can trigger a case of PD. Another simple way to start a case of PD is to sit for a long time while the crotch of the pants ride up tightly and apply pressure to the genitals. All of these examples show how fragile the tunica albuginea of the penis can be at times. With this in mind it would seem foolish to deliberately apply any kind of massage force to the penis in treating PD. Therefore, never underestimate the sensitivity of the tunica layer of the penis. For this reason all massage is delivered to the tissue around the genital area but never on it.

One of the primary reasons that massage can be so universally effective in a wide range of health problems is that it assists the movement of lymphatic fluid generally throughout the body, and most specifically in the target area of the diseased tissue. Before we get into the technique it would be good to review a little background to explain why increasing lymphatic flow is so important in treating PD, and many other disease processes.

First, you must understand a few things about the lymphatic system of your body. The lymphatic system can be compared to the sewer system of your home. The sewer system has an enclosed network of pipes that drain fluid from your home to be purified elsewhere. The lymphatic system also has an enclosed system of lymphatic vessels that are similar to veins, which carry fluid to the liver for purification. The fluid in the lymphatic vessels is called "lymph."

More lymph fluid is found in the body than blood; the average person has about 6.2 liters of lymph fluid and "only" 5 liters of blood.

Every part of the body has a blood and lymph supply; blood and lymph go into and out of every body tissue and area of the body. If the lymphatic fluid does not flow freely into and out of an area, then the blood will also not flow freely since the two systems are indirectly connected. We have all heard of lymph nodes. These are the little bean shaped nodules or "filters" placed along the course of the lymph vessels that remove toxins, bacteria and dead cells from the body. The lymph nodes are found all over the body and are usually unnoticeable. If an infection starts in any part of the body, the lymph nodes in that area enlarge and become painful to touch as they begin to collect and swell with toxins and dead tissue cells.

When these lymph nodes become swollen and inflamed, while they assist the body to fight an infection, congestion can occur in the lymph node resulting in general swelling of the entire area. This is a common situation when severe inflammation is present in the body. When the flow of lymph becomes reduced for any reason, this results in a reduced capacity to defend against disease, and impaired tissue repair and healing. In these cases of reduced lymphatic flow the tissue becomes filled and swollen with lymph fluid and it is called edema.

Massage is used to increase lymphatic movement and promote tissue fluid drainage, to assure good movement of blood and nutrients into and out of every part of the body, as well as removal of tissue toxins that are given off continuously during normal cellular activity. These functions of the lymphatic system make it particularly important in the treatment of PD. If the lymphatic system of the lower pelvis is not working fully, then blood flow in and out of that same region of the body will also be limited; nutrients cannot enter, and toxins cannot leave adequately. Any area of the body can heal more rapidly when the lymph fluid flows properly, allowing the blood to enter and toxins to exit more freely.

The massage discussed in this section is not the gentle or relaxing variety of massage given to the top layers of tissue or muscles. This massage is aggressive, deep, and very often a little uncomfortable, verging on painful, if it is to do you and your PD any good. How deep and aggressive the massage is delivered depends on personal tolerance and motivation. You will note that during the actual time of massage the pain level can be quite high, but as soon as the pressure is stopped, so is the discomfort. In this way you will know that you are delivering the right amount of pressure and force. If the pain and discomfort continue after your fingertips have been removed from the area, then you are being unnecessarily forceful and aggressive. Also, you will know if you are overdoing it if you notice bruise marks on yourself the next day. If you are going too deep, merely lighten up the next time.

NOTE: **Do not massage the actual PD scar or the penis**. Do not apply force or pressure to the penis; work around the genitals, in the immediate area of the groin and lower pelvis. If you massage or bruise the PD scar you run the risk of injury to the penis and tunica albuginea, possibly injuring this tissue again and further increasing the PD scar.

Technique:

1. Lie on your back, bend both knees, keep feet flat on bed or floor, and spread legs apart at the groin to make a 90° angle between the right and left thigh. Your two legs are now perpendicular to each other.

2. Relax the muscles to allow for deep fingertip pressure through the lower abdominal wall and groin area down to pelvic bone, and the deep muscle and tendon layers and related soft tissue.

3. Use fingertip pressure of about 3-4 pounds, maybe 5-6 pounds or so, if you have a very large or heavy abdomen.

4. Slowly and gently press down to the front portion of the pelvic bone – under pubic hair area – in an area approximately 4" top to bottom X 12" across left to right. Work over the inguinal area or groin crease that is found on each side of the pelvis where the tops of the thigh bones connect to it, just lateral to the pubic hair.

5. Using this 3-4 pounds, or so, of fingertip pressure, locate areas more uncomfortable to touch than other adjacent tissue. **Stay off the penis, and do not contact or massage the PD scar.**

6. When you locate an area of contracted and tight tissue, you will note that the same fingertip pressure that was nicely comfortable in other neighboring tissue of the pelvis will suddenly cause discomfort you did not feel in other areas – the same amount of pressure causes some areas to really hurt badly and others do not hurt at all.

7. There should be no difference in the amount of pressure or force that you use; the difference in an area that hurts and one that doesn't should be based on the basic sensitivity and soreness of the tissue you are touching. **You are trying to locate tissue that is already sensitive; you are not trying to make it sensitive or bruised by using excessive force.**

8. Stay on each sensitive area discovered for 20-30 seconds. If you keep about the same level of pressure on this sensitive tissue, you will have about the same level of discomfort.

9. While you maintain this same pressure, slowly rub the spot in a very small circular or side-to-side motion that is perhaps ¼ to ½ inch in size. This motion should not make your fingertips slide on the skin; your fingertips do not move on the skin, but you are slightly moving the tissue below the surface in a small area of massage under your fingertips.

10. If you find many closely placed sore and tender areas in a small region, then concentrate on those which are the worst.

11. You will note that almost always the sore areas will feel different from non-sore areas (lumpy, bumpy, hard, dense, stringy, ropey, raised, ridged and all together different from the soft and pliable tissue that does not hurt).

12. When you find an area of different contour, density or elevation, examine it with your fingertips in a variety of directions and angles to locate the particular direction that causes unique discomfort or pain sensation. You will be surprised at the different contours and density of tissue, and you will find these reactions and physical qualities change from day to day.

13. A painful area will almost always have a different contour, density or elevation than another area that is not sore to the touch just a fraction of an inch away. Important areas to treat will often feel much lumpier than others, have a sharp ridge or well-defined margin; most feel like a tight guitar string laying in deep tissue or just on top of the pelvic bone.

14. After a few days of the pressure, rubbing, stroking, and digging into the painful nodules of the soft tissue, you will notice these areas will feel slightly different to the touch – less lumpy or bumpy, less elevated, less painful, or softer; perhaps a previous sharp ridge or guitar string formation will feel duller, less well defined and more relaxed.

15. You should not feel bruised or sore to the touch after you are finished massaging an area – if you do, you are working too aggressively; lighten your touch.

Do not attempt to make huge changes in this tissue in a day or two by working very hard and deep – that strategy does not work well. The idea is go slowly and steadily over a period of time – perhaps a few weeks – to make the best changes possible. You will actually accomplish more with less force. Continue doing this kind of deep soft tissue massage until all painful and lumpy, bumpy, nodular and stringy formations are gone.

By working these areas of tight contracted soft tissue you will do a tremendous amount of good to increase the lymphatic flow and therefore the blood flow in the lower pelvis. This is an important way to provide a great advantage over PD.

Exercise for PD

There are only two kinds of exercise that a person can do to get stronger: isotonic exercise and isometric exercise.

Isotonic exercise is the kind that is usually thought of when exercise is mentioned, like weightlifting, chopping wood or running. For an isotonic exercise to occur three important things must happen:

1. The muscles being used or exercised will change length, meaning the muscles will shorten during the contraction phase of the activity.

2. The body part being exercised will move, as when doing push-ups, walking, or fixing your car.

3. The strength of the muscle contraction involved in the exercise or work being done is variable, sometimes great and sometimes very little.

Isometric exercise is different in several key ways. You seldom do an isometric exercise unless you are involved in extremely heavy work that causes complete muscle overload. It is possible for some people to go for months without ever doing an isometric activity. But, let's say you are a plumber. You attempt to loosen a tight fitting on a pipe that has been rusted over. You pull on the wrench as absolutely hard as you can, but nothing happens. Your face gets red, your arms and body tremble from the effort, but the nut does not loosen and the wrench and your arms do not move. That is an isometric activity. For an isometric exercise to occur three important things must happen:

1. The muscles being used will not change length, meaning the muscles do not shorten.

2. The body part being exercised will not move, as when trying to turn a door knob when the door is locked, or trying to lift a refrigerator by yourself; in spite of your effort, nothing moves.

3. The strength of the muscle contraction involved in the exercise or work being done must be constant and it must be the maximum contraction of which you are capable. A half-effort or a weak effort is not an isometric activity. This is a critical point that will be stressed several times as we discuss treatment for PD.

Ever heard of a Kegel exercise? A Kegel exercise is simply an isometric (full force, no movement) exercise of the one particular muscle of the lower pelvis.

If you have heard of the Kegel exercise it was probably in relation to treatment of a woman's urinary problem. Kegel exercises are prescribed routinely for a wide variety of woman's urinary problems, even frequent bladder infection. This gets back to the need for increased blood supply and lymphatic drainage in a wide variety of problems, even bacterial infection.

Benefits a man can receive from doing Kegel exercises:

1. Increase the blood flow to the genital area, and so support sexual arousal mechanisms.

2. Increase blood flow and lymphatic drainage to the genitals to facilitate healing of a wide variety of health problems, such as Peyronie's disease.

3. Strengthen the muscles that are used in ejaculation. Men who Kegel gain greater control over the timing of ejaculation. The PC muscle is the muscle that involuntary "pumps" when you ejaculate. Strengthening the PC muscle – and learning to control it – may help to control and delay ejaculation in men. With this skill a man can have an orgasm and still not ejaculate, enabling him to have multiple orgasms. See, this is a very important section after all, isn't it?!

4. Kegel exercises prevent urinary incontinence and other problems often associated with aging.

However, men can also benefit from doing Kegel exercises for the variety of different reasons listed above, the most important one of which is PD. The entire interest in Kegel exercises has to do with the particular muscle that is involved, and is a special way of strengthening the lower pelvic muscles, specifically the pubococcygeus (PC) muscle, which is a sling-shaped muscle that surrounds your anus and prostate gland.

The PC muscle lies between the hip bones in the lower pelvic area. At the bottom of the pelvis, several layers of muscle stretch between your legs. The muscles attach to the front, back, and sides of the pelvis at the level of the anus. This will explain why when you begin in a few minutes to do a Kegel exercise for the first time, you will notice that mostly you will contract the anus muscles.

Ever make yourself stop urinating before you were done? The PC muscle is the muscle you used to do it. To locate PC: while urinating, stop and start the stream several times. If you cannot do this, or have difficulty in "finding" it to stop the flow of urine, or you have a problem with urinary or anal leaking, you really need this exercise.

Here's how to get started: Next time when you have the urge to urinate, sit on the toilet with your feet and legs spread apart, start to urinate, then stop the flow. Practice stopping and restarting several times. The muscle you are using is the PC.

It usually takes several attempts to actually isolate the PC muscle – as was mentioned earlier, the anal and buttock muscles have a tendency to actually get involved, so it is necessary to keep the legs wide apart while you are still learning the control you need. After you have familiarized yourself with the sensation of contracting the PC muscle, it is time to practice holding the contractions. First try holding a contraction for several seconds three or four times during different times of the day. Over several days you can gradually increase the time until you are holding it for about eight seconds. If you can hold it for longer than eight seconds that is great, but is not necessary for our purposes.

Kegel Exercise Technique

To be done correctly and develop strength promptly, follow these rules for doing a Kegel exercise:

1. Maximum contraction force – total effort, can't do it any harder, no half effort will result in the kind of strength gain you are looking to develop.

2. Hold the contraction for 8 seconds; relax 8 seconds.

3. Do exercises in "sets" or groups.

   • MAXIMUM contraction of PC muscles as hard as you can. (If you are doing an isometric contraction of your fist you will have the knuckles go white and the hand will tremble.) When you are doing a Kegel exercise, you will want to contract the PC muscle just as hard. Initially, you will not feel like much is happening down there, because of the relative weakness of the PC when you get started. After a week or two of these exercises, you will begin to feel a greater level of strength and awareness of this area.

   • To time your isometric contractions, try counting the seconds by mentally saying to yourself at a normal speaking pace : 1000 **one,** 1000 **two,** 1000 **three,** 1000 **four,** 1000 **five,** 1000 **six,** 1000 **seven,** 1000 **eigh**t. This will take eight seconds from start to finish.

   • **Example of "3 Rep" series of Kegel exercises:**

   Set One: 1. Maximum contraction 8 seconds, rest 8 seconds.

                   2. Maximum contraction 8 seconds, rest 8 seconds.

                   3. Maximum contraction 8 seconds.

                   Rest: 20-30 seconds

Set Two: 1. Maximum contraction 8 seconds, rest 8 seconds.

2. Maximum contraction 8 seconds, rest 8 seconds.

3. Maximum contraction 8 seconds.

Rest: 20-30 seconds

Set Three: 1. Maximum contraction 8 seconds, rest 8 seconds.

2. Maximum contraction 8 seconds, rest 8 seconds.

3. Maximum contraction 8 seconds.

Stop. You are done until you do this again in 2-3 days.

Do this group of three sets three times the first week – maybe even the first two weeks if these exercises make you feel tired or sore in the lower pelvis. When you no longer feel tired or sore from doing the three sets of exercises, then increase the number of contractions in a set from three to four (go from a 3 rep to a 4 rep set, three times), for a week or two. Of course, if the basic set of three repetitions makes you sore you can do less and then slowly build up from there.

Set One: 1. Maximum contraction 8 seconds, rest 8 seconds.

2. Maximum contraction 8 seconds, rest 8 seconds.

3. Maximum contraction 8 seconds, rest 8 seconds.

4. Maximum contraction 8 seconds.

Rest: 20-30 seconds

Sets Two and Three, Same as Set One

After you are doing the increased number of contractions with no problem, then increase the number of contractions you do in a set from four to five (go from a 4 rep set to a 5 rep set, three times), for a week or two.

Slowly increase the number of contractions in a set, but do not do more than three sets. The goal is to get to three sets with each set consisting of 10 maximum contractions (a 10 rep set, three times, for a total of 30 maximum contractions).

When you get up to three sets of 10 full maximum contractions in a session, you might consider additional PC muscle exercises. This next level of pelvic muscle exercise is simply a variation of the Kegel, in which you briefly give the same PC muscle a hard quick squeeze in a pumping action – not the usual full maximum 8-second contraction – in a long series of these short contractions. Do this series of short fast contractions at the end of the usual three sets of Kegel exercise so your PC muscle is warmed up and ready for this heavier use.

To do a rapid series of bursts of contraction of the PC, simply give the PC a good hard squeeze, rest just long enough to get ready for another good hard squeeze, and then another, and so on. You should be able to easily do one contraction a second. No contraction is held, but is simply tightened and then immediately relaxed. Start out by rapidly tightening and immediately letting the PC relax about 25 times.

If you do this rapid fire exercise series of 25 contractions at the end of a full isometric session of three sets of 10 contractions, you will likely feel a little tired in the lower pelvis. Again be sure to do this exercise series no more than three times a week.

After a week or two, if you feel no soreness or fatigue at the end of the last session, try going up to 50 rapid-fire contractions of the PC at the end of your standard isometric exercises. The goal is to get up to 250 such rapid-fire contractions of the PC.

This kind of heavy exercise program for the PC will take about 10-12 minutes to perform. It will greatly increase the circulation to the lower pelvis, with the added health benefit of improved circulation to the prostate gland.

Like any other exercise, it is important to rest any muscle you exercise to give it a chance to recover and rebuild so that strength can be gained during the recovery phase. Therefore, daily Kegel exercise is not recommended at any time, even when you are first starting out. Kegel exercises three times a week is sufficient for a good program.

- When doing Kegels, notice when your abdominal muscles or your anal muscles feel like they also want to join in the exercise. Pay attention that these muscles are not used, only the PD. When you are doing it properly, a small region near the scrotum should feel like it is being used and the scrotum will elevate slightly.

- When you are skilled at Kegel exercises you will be able to do them without anyone knowing you are doing them... on the train, in the barber chair, at boring meetings at work, while watching TV, at red lights, and other times during the day all become opportunities to work quietly on improving your sexual health!

Using a series of both sustained and brief Kegel contractions faithfully, perhaps for the rest of your life, should enable you to make great progress in your PD treatment plan and keep your prostate healthier.

Chapter 9 – PD Can Be a Family Affair, Unfortunately

Ω - **To live a better life, be happier and healthier in spite of your PD, and increase your chance of successfully treating it …**

… you must be content in your personal and family life. PD destroys families and tests the love of those around you. More than at any other time in his life, the man with PD needs those same people whom he is pushing away in anger, frustration and shame. It is a bad time for anyone who is in the pathway of PD. Allow this chapter to open some areas of personal reflection and family discussion – learn to talk openly about this problem so that you can also heal the inner wounds.

Perhaps the Greatest Tragedy of PD

Most family and interpersonal problems that occur because of PD often continue to extreme and heartbreaking conclusions. No person, male or female, and no family can be adequately prepared for the deep conflicts that develop as a direct and indirect result of PD. More than just overwhelming, tragic events, and tensions can develop for two primary reasons within a family that experiences PD. The first is that an abundance of questions and only a few rare answers surround so many important issues. And the second is since PD is a disease so few are able to talk about, it is easy for the personal plight to escalate when shrouded in a atmosphere of shame, guilt and embarrassment.

In one way or another PD pushes and pulls at the total family structure, without exception, in ways that can be obvious or subtle. The multiple layers of stress that arise in a family swell up out of the frustration and confusion from the many unknown and variable aspects of PD. All levels of family life can be affected; problems and stresses filter through from the primary issue of PD and multiply their influence in all areas of family life. Not just sexual activity is affected by the presence of PD in a family; all levels of a marriage and family structure are stressed. Any problems in a marriage that already existed before the PD will likely be intensified to near the breaking point, and often beyond.

A committed couple, when instructed and prepared, can be made stronger by the test that is posed by PD. If a man is lucky enough to have his physical problem dealt with properly, as well as his interpersonal problems also addressed adequately, his relationship can benefit. The onset of PD becomes a real test of character for each individual involved; additionally, it becomes a test of their compatibility as a couple and their combined communication and problem solving skills. As with so many problems that occur in a life, PD can ruin or strengthen the individuals involved.

Anger and Frustration

One reason in particular stands out to explain PD's damaging effect on a relationship and marriage. While certainly many other reasons exist, the most corrupting influences on interpersonal bonds come from the increased levels of anger and frustration that are found in a PD family. Even with men who are otherwise slow to anger, generally easy going and gentle souls, a unique button is pushed in PD. It is as though a personality change occurs that centers on the display of anger and frustration. A higher level of anger than usual is brought to the surface in almost all cases of PD I have encountered, and it is more easily and more frequently triggered than usual. Men who previously never yelled at their spouses will do so, and those who on occasion had displays of "average" anger suddenly behave like a cornered animal who strikes out wildly toward those who attempt to help him.

It seems that a man's frustration level is so burdened by PD that anger is uncharacteristically elevated. From all I have heard and seen, it appears to be a widespread phenomenon that runs very deep in PD. Men with whom I have talked about this phenomenon admit, "I don't know what comes over me, I really can't control my anger. It's like I am someone else." Add to this volatile situation a wife who has problems of her own dealing with PD, and it is easy to understand how major marital distress can erupt. Life, while dealing with elevated levels of anger and frustration, can be difficult in the PD family.

Communicating with Your Spouse

No easy answer comes to mind for the question, "What can I do to keep PD from ruining my marriage?" Each marriage has a unique set of dynamics and unspoken rules by which it operates and survives. Each couple will solve – or not solve – their PD problem in their own unique way. Additionally, no set rules can be followed in these cases since there are no set problem patterns that develop in PD. Some men become impotent, some become argumentative, and others just sulk; these different problems require unique strategic responses.

In one marriage, the greatest aspect of the PD problem might be the mistrust a husband with PD feels toward his wife, because she had been unfaithful previously – this would not exist in a family with no history of marital infidelity. In another marriage, the greatest aspect of the PD problem might be the shame and disgust a man feels about the distorted appearance of his penis, because of childhood sexual abuse he carries deep within him even to today. And in yet another family situation, the greatest aspect of the PD problem might be guilt that a man feels because of his inability to provide sexual satisfaction to a wife. With so many ways the PD experience can play out in a family, the web of stresses and problems are countless and complex and so are the responses.

From my observations, these are the common qualities and shared strengths of those who survive as a couple, in spite of PD:

- Open communication
- Problem solvers, not problem stirrers
- Commitment to making the best of a bad situation
- Ability to forgive, forget and move forward
- Adaptability

While I am not a marriage counselor, I am someone who has dealt with patients and their many problems for almost 40 years. From my experience in dealing with the unique marital discord that develops because of PD, very often no good answer can be provided for the intense personal tensions that eventually arise within a PD family. This is so because far more questions than answers confound the problem solving process; it is difficult to resolve a crisis when most of the discussions end with "I don't know," and "I can't."

With PD, every marital problem seems to avoid a simple or complete answer, but only conclude with a meager compromise that is unfair to one or both partners. The best option to a PD problem is usually one that is least objectionable or unfair to the fewest people. Often these solutions are discovered by simply asking many questions and facing the uncomfortable answers squarely and honestly. In this light, sometimes the best a person can do to solve a large marital problem is to review all possible answers while weighing the value of each as a potential compromise.

Often, problem-solving in PD is simply a matter of selecting "the lesser of many evils." While attempting to address the many Peyronie's disease questions and problems that arise, the best answer often turns out to be a non-solution that is finally accepted not because it is brilliant, insightful and fair, but simply because it is the best of other bad options. To discover these best of the undesirable options, all options and compromises must be seriously considered. By evaluating an option that would not have been given a second thought before PD, it now becomes a possibility that would not otherwise have been considered. In the face of a catastrophe everything changes and a person does what is necessary for survival. PD can be like that. From the range of possible options, the one chosen is often no more than the least offensive compromise that both partners can tolerate. It might not seem fair, that no one is truly delighted with a particular solution, but that is the nature of compromise. Perfection doesn't enter into the discussion. Compromise and tolerance become the standard. Admittedly, it takes very big people to do this and some couples never learn to compromise and tolerate the changes that are forced on them. Bit, if you are serious about saving your marriage, you must.

The worst scenario usually occurs when one or both partners assume that a genuinely great answer – a perfect solution that leaves everyone happy because it is brilliant in so many ways – is somewhere to be found. This is fantasy in the world

109

of PD. They look and look for a perfect answer, and it is no where to be found. Each looks to have the other partner make some sacrifice or change that will cause all of the problems to suddenly disappear. Often this never happens. Dissatisfaction and more anger can only result when problems become worse, and sprout up in new areas of their relationship.

In those cases in which the couple will not accept compromise as a solution, and this is a large segment unfortunately, their misery continues to grow and it pulls them further apart. Some couples do not have sufficient compassion and understanding for each other and refuse to cooperate in a spirit of compromise. They would rather fight than do what is needed to get along.

Though it is regrettable that couples are put into this terrible situation, peace and harmony arrive with the ability to compromise and accept less than a perfect situation. Less tolerant couples, being unable to select the least offensive compromise between two or three undesirable choices, and "learn to live with it," escalate their problems and separate from each other.

Other couples create a positive atmosphere of compromise and tolerance for the limits of the other, and they work things out. They grow as individuals and they grow as a loving and functioning marital unit. They do not fight the unfairness and inevitable limitations of PD. They do not focus on what used to be, but they squarely and bravely face what is. The woman is usually the strong one initially, and she inspires the man to see his situation differently. They learn to play the cards dealt to them, and so eventually develop a better marriage for it.

PDI does not for a moment suggest giving in to PD, or quitting, or doing only what is easy – no, not at all. What is suggested is that while on the one hand you compromise the best possible solutions to your problems with your mate, on the other hand you fight mightily against this disease by using all of the aggressive conservative tactics that **PDI** is known for. **PDI** suggests that you come together as a couple, being as soft, forgiving, understanding, and loving toward each other, to helping each other trough the problems of PD, and at the same time declare total war on the real enemy that has attacked your marriage.

Adding Fuel to the Fire

Everyone knows of people who are their own worst enemies in times of crisis. They do not handle stress well, any stress; they fall apart in troubled times. They make matters worse for themselves by not thinking clearly or behaving maturely; they make bad decisions. In the case of PD, it is common for a man – especially the man – to contribute to his family stress by inappropriate and exaggerated behavior in a wide variety of ways. Is that possible with you? Are you making matters worse than they need to be by how you are handling yourself and your problem? Are you adding fuel to your own fire?

Is this to suggest that PD is only a minor inconvenience that can be shrugged off like a flat tire on a rainy day? No, not at all. I have come to understand that in spite of my own best intentions I was causing my marriage unintended stresses while not realizing it. A few times I think I came closer to falling apart emotionally than at any time in my life. It was scary. It made me stop and wonder _what I was allowing_ to happen to myself. I did not want to lose control of myself like that, and refused to give in to the blind anger that I felt so deeply. I simply did not give myself permission to go so close to the edge ever again. And it worked for me. You must figure out your personal control mechanism. You must not allow yourself to wallow in self-pity, disgust, hopelessness, anger, humiliation or any of the forms your demons can take on. You must not allow PD to destroy you or what you own.

In the beginning anger and denial rule, but eventually it must stop. Do not wallow in it and allow it to fester. Outbursts of rage, while understandable, must be controlled in appropriate ways. Your righteous anger must be followed by positive and constructive action – a time for sober determination. The outbursts must be rare, directed away from loved ones, and perhaps kept as a totally private luxury to release the demons that grow inside. Each person will follow his own path away from the confusion and anger, hopefully leading to a better place of personal peace and growth.

Only those who have lived through the PD experience can really appreciate the unique personal hardships that develop. Each man with PD will react differently to the stress of PD because of his unique personality, previous life experiences, and his own balance of strengths and weaknesses. When PD happens to someone, he usually reveals what lies beneath the surface and he merely becomes more of what he was before the problem began. As a point of reflection and opportunity to "fix your leaking boat," here are just some of the possible emotions that come out of the lowest point that PD can take a man.

- Moodiness and anger about PD
- Withdrawal and lack of communication – isolation from your mate because you don't know what else to do
- Frustration with lack of medical information and help
- Feeling ugly and freakish
- Feeling less masculine, less confident of being able to maintain respect and a husbandly position in your marriage
- Vulnerable and inferior to other men who have no sexual problem
- Shame and humiliation because of distortion
- Insecure because of lost virility
- Silly and ashamed that you did this to yourself by masturbation or a secret sexual practice that you are not proud of
- Unworthiness because of inability to be good sexual partner

- Unworthiness because you know that if the tables were turned, you could not be as big and kind a person to her as she is being to you

- Pride is being tested because you have never had to be on the receiving end of sorrow and pity; you are not accustomed to being the one who has the problem; your pride is hurt because now it is official, you are flawed and uniquely imperfect

- Anger that she was one who injured your penis, she started the whole PD mess because she was careless and awkward

- Anger that you can recall no trauma or injury to penis, that you did nothing to develop this problem

- Anger about lost sexual expression and pleasurable part of life

- Guilt that you actually did something stupid to ruin your life and your wife's life

- Reminds you of sexual abuse that occurred in childhood, and you are feeling old problems of abuse from the past in addition to other feelings because of the PD.

- Penis looking weird and grotesque feeds your feeling of deep inferiority that comes from the way you were raised, making you feel worthless and ashamed

A lot of bad memories and forgotten problems from the past can resurface because of PD. These then can combine with all the new problems of PD. Taken together, it is common to experience new levels of anger and frustration never experienced previously. So when she says to you, "What is bothering you?" it is difficult to know where and how to begin explaining it all. Many men find it safer and easier to just say nothing, and withdraw. This is a huge mistake, often fatal to a marriage. Withdrawal solves nothing and distances you from her at a time you should be drawing together.

Her viewpoint

Has your wife complained in the past that you do not communicate sufficiently for her? Please notice how that question is asked, "sufficiently for her."

Women have different needs, much greater needs, to communicate than men's needs. Not only do they have an actual need to communicate to those in their social group, the more important you are to her the more her need to connect on a personal level with you – often. On top of that, when someone in her social group is in trouble, the need to connect with that person increases. For her it is not just something to do, it is not a preference, it is not a weakness to babble on and on, nor is it something that can be omitted or limited without consequences.

Burn this into your testosterone brain: Women actually possess a **need** to talk to those people who are close to them. The closer and more important the person in their lives, the greater the vital need to communicate often, and on a deep and intimate level. Since you can assume you have a fairly high place in your spouse's social group, she really needs to talk to you.

It is almost a cliché: "He just doesn't talk to me anymore." It is spoken and written about so often that the words do not seem important from sheer repetition. In movies, in jokes, in magazines, in conversations, in television stories: One woman is talking to another, and says. "Oh, my husband! I don't know what I am going to do with him! He just won't talk to me. Talking to him is like talking to a brick wall. He just won't open up." On and on she goes. We have all heard this kind of dialogue before. To a man it sounds like the woman is just complaining about something small and unimportant. But read between the lines, interject your deeper understanding that she is truly referring to the fact that her husband is not fulfilling a vital real-life need of hers – not just to gossip and chit-chat – but to enter into a special bonding experience that is similar to sex for a man. With this insight you are in a better position to really understand what she has been asking for, and you probably denying to her.

That kind of dialogue is not much different than a locker room conversation in which one man is saying to his sympathetic buddy, "Man, I don't know what I am going to do about my wife! It is driving me crazy! She just won't have sex with me like I need it. Having sex with her is like having sex with a dead fish. She just doesn't warm up." On and on he goes. It is really the same thing in both examples: Deep, powerful, basic, primitive needs that are not being met by a partner.

Communication Is More Important Than You Know

Since your marriage is already under stress from PD, depriving her of this second fundamental need to communicate with you (the first basic need for her is sex), is a further denial she might find intolerable. It can be so unsettling to her emotionally that it jeopardizes her feelings for you and marriage to you. If you deny her access to your personal side, while at the same time she is not receiving the sexual closeness she also needs, you might take her to a point of isolation from you that jeopardizes your total relationship with her. With the additional stress of PD in your marriage, she just might feel so neglected, isolated, and unfulfilled that she looks elsewhere for both of her needs to be met. You could force her to respond to your perceived rejection of her, by her own rejection of you. If this happens, you should now understand how you contribute to this problem by simply not opening up and communicating with her about your problem. It's that important to her.

You might think you are communicating with her sufficiently, but it is a good bet that you are wrong about how well you are doing. She probably needs more. If she has been telling you all along that you do not talk to her, hopefully this discussion will help you to understand her on a different level. For many women the need to simply talk to the people who are important to them is a deep primitive need; it can be similar, and sometimes just as intense, as a man's need for sexual release. Think of it in these terms: She might need sex once a week and you need sex once a day. She thinks, "I'm doing it enough, I did it last week," and you are thinking "She is

113

holding out on me, I need it once a day." She doesn't understand your need because she is basing her evaluation of your sexual needs by her standards, not yours. It is the same with a woman's need to communicate. You think, "I told her once last month how I feel, that should be enough," and she is thinking, "He is holding out on me, I need it once a day."

It's true: Sex is for men, like communication is for women. It's weird, I know. But doesn't it explain a lot of her behavior, what you have seen and heard, what she has told you over and over again? Look at it from her standpoint: Why should it be so terribly important that men ejaculate all the time? OK. It feels good, and all that. But the male need for sex goes beyond the obvious physical pleasure and satisfaction. It is a deep and nameless primitive urge that is difficult to discuss, and can only be understood when it is felt. It is an urgency that comes from somewhere in the lower part of the brain that drives men simply and impulsively to want to procreate.

A woman has a similar feeling in her need to keep her group, her tribe, her small band of family together. It is her way of making sure she multiplies her number; if the group communicates it stands a better chance to survive and multiply.

That's it: Talking, communicating with her close people, staying united with her "tribe" is a survival strategy for her, just as much as the need for frequent and widespread sexual conquest is for you. It is a need that is wired into her brain, much the same way the need for intercourse is wired into the male brain. It gives her a high, a place of comfort and security; it makes her feel good – just like sex. She is fulfilling a need a man does not experience or understand.

If you are concerned only about her need for sexual satisfaction, you are fulfilling only part of her needs. You are missing the point that by not communicating with your mate, you are now depriving her of two things that she needs from you: sexual satisfaction and communication. Of these, perhaps in her case, the second might actually be more important and stronger than the first. It is a huge mistake to not understand this. She can forgive you for the first, because she realizes your penis has a significant problem. But she cannot forgive you for the second because even though you can still listen and talk, you are not listening to her as she tries once again to explain this other great need she has. You will lose her in spite of her love for you, because she is feeling neglected, abused, misunderstood and unloved. You will lose her because you are not fulfilling this basic and primitive need that she has to communicate with you. Yes, it is that important.

A huge problem comes about when the man does not help his mate fulfill that need, just as if the woman does not fulfill the sexual need for her man. She feels disconnected in a way that a man does not experience or understand, and she feels that her place in his life is threatened. Not a good feeling for her. If threatened in this way, she will likely think of going somewhere else where she can feel safe, secure and protected with another mate – since this is what the talking and personal sharing is all about. It is simple and straightforward, and makes sense from the standpoint of the basic urges and needs all people possess.

Can you see how the male and female are doing something similar, but using different means to the same end of keeping the tribe going?

Once you get this idea, once you understand the need, once you know what is driving her great interest in finding out how your day went or what you are feeling, then you can come closer to improving your relationship. If you have a successful marriage, it is very likely that she has already done her part in raising her sexual response to meet your needs – even though she might not experience them in the same way you do or understand them. Now it is your turn to raise your communication response to meet her needs. It is only fair, and it is what will help immeasurably to make you both happier with each other and perhaps save your marriage.

If you are wise, and use your understanding of how deep and vital this need to communicate is for her, your relationship will flourish in spite of PD. It can be the secret that makes you a better husband and lover than all others. It is all or a good part of the answer to much of your previous and current marital problems, and it can guide you through the many problems that might arise because of PD.

Taking Care of All Her Needs

If you are feeling vulnerable, threatened, weak, and less than the virile man you once were, and worry that since you cannot perform sexually as you once did, you might be replaced. If this is a concern for you, it is because you do not understand the entire dynamic of what motivates a woman.

As the distress increases and the problems worsen for the person she cares about (you), she is made to live with a disturbing problem in her social group and this makes her feel ill at ease. Her response is an ever-increasing need to communicate and share deeper feelings with that person. She needs, really needs like taking a breath, for you to open up and simply talk to her. If you do, if you meet her communication need, she will be far more likely and far more generous and forgiving for not meeting her other need of sex. Meeting two out of two needs would increase your bonds of love and friendship; one out of two is good; none out of two could be disastrous.

To secure your relationship with your wife, to make your marriage less vulnerable because of your sexual limit and loss, at least address any communication problem that you might have. You owe it to your wife, and your marriage, to think of her need to communicate with you about your problem. Depriving her of your participation and involvement in this other fundamental need she has can be so disheartening and unsettling that it jeopardizes her feelings about you and marriage to you.

Opening up

You might think you have explained enough about what is happening to you since your PD started. After all, you told her once about what the PD was like and how you were embarrassed, didn't you? That should be enough for her, because you know it would be enough for you, right? That is judging her need on the basis of your need. We already established that this does not work and that it is not fair to her.

If you told her what is going on in your head and your heart, of your fears, and your attitudes about yourself, did you tell her all of it? Have you really told her everything, or are you still holding back? Are you telling a part of what you feel and know? Have you held back certain uncomfortable ideas and feelings that are just so private or painful that you cannot express them?

Perhaps you are just more private and quiet than the average person. And perhaps she has higher than average need to talk about things that are important to her, maybe even to the point of endless discussion of things that have been explored continuously. That is something the two of you will have to work out together. But the important issue is that you take the initiative to make changes in you that will show greater awareness and improved concern for her need to communicate. If you can modify your behavior based on her need to talk, she should be able to modify her behavior based on your needs as a quiet person. You come together in the middle at a satisfactory level of compromise. Not perfect, perhaps, but better than either of you were doing before. This is the basis of a better marriage and one that grows deeper and stronger together because of PD, not destroyed by it.

Do Any of These Apply to You?

Your communication issue should be receptive to change and improvement. If they are not, then you must decide why not.

- Are you communicating less since getting PD? Why?

- Are you communicating less to protect yourself? From what?

- Are you quiet because of shame and humiliation?

- Are you pouting? That's OK. I understanding pouting. I pouted often and loudly when I first got PD; I was a champion pouter. I didn't know what else to do, so I pouted. When pouting didn't work, I had full blown-temper tantrums like a little child. It made matters worse. I am lucky to have a wife who loves me enough to tolerate my nonsense for a while, and then she laid down the law. She straightened me out as only a wife can do, and I was smart enough to listen to her. Once again she helped me tremendously, and we are now closer because of it.

- Are you communicating less to hurt her? Why? What is so important from your past that you should ruin your future?

116

- If you are <u>involuntarily</u> depriving her of sexual activity, why are you <u>voluntarily</u> depriving her further of her need to communicate? Can you see how this is a double-unfairness to her and a needless injury to someone you love?

- What have you told her about how you feel about your PD problem and what it is doing to you inside? Was it honest and complete?

- Can you explain how you feel in your heart, and what is going on inside your head?

- What have you really told her? What would you like to tell her that you cannot bring yourself to say?

- What can you do to better communicate with her?

The questions can easily continue on, but the answers are very hard to come by. There are no answers that can be given here that would accurately apply to everyone. So the best we can do is to ask a lot of questions and wait for the still small voice from within that sometimes shouts an answer so loudly that it cannot be avoided. This is a good thing. I hope you are listening.

Be honest with yourself, and her. Make her feel included with you in all levels of your problem, as she <u>needs</u> to be. Do not hurt your woman by keeping her out of your life. She actually needs to help you. You will lose her, and it will be your entire fault for being too weak and afraid to be honest. Be man enough to take care of this need for her.

Questions to ponder and areas to think about:

- What have you told her about how you feel? Really told her? What have you held back when you were trying to talk to her?

- Do you fear you are going to lose her to another man? Have you told her this?

- Do you fear she will be tempted to go to other men for sexual satisfaction?

- Do you fear losing your home and marriage?

- Do you hate the idea that you are responsible for hurting your wife?

- Do you fear losing her respect and admiration?

- Do you fear you are seen as less than a total man?

- Do you feel like you are cheating her?

- Are you embarrassed about the way that you look?

- Do you feel like she is thinking about cheating on you because you can no longer be the man you once were?

117

- With the onset of PD do you feel like you have lost a trusted friend, your comforter, and source of personal pleasure?

- Do you feel a loss of personal pride by looking less sexually attractive?

- Do you think you must be ugly to her?

- Do you fear and hate feeling more vulnerable and beholding to your wife's sympathy and feeling sorry for you?

- Do you hate it because you feel like she is feeling pity for you?

- Does it bother you that others might talk about your problem if they were ever to find out about it somehow?

- Does it make you feel threatened to be the subject of jokes and speculation about how badly your PD has affected you?

- Do you feel like you are going to explode in a rage over the unfairness of this whole disease that no one seems to understand?

- Do you feel helpless to get your life back together like it was?

- Do you feel humiliated because you think you look like a freak?

- Are you angry that you did nothing wrong and you got this problem that is ruining the life that you enjoyed?

- Are you angry about losing the ability to engage in sex like before?

- Do you feel deep sorrow about the loss of important part of your life?

- How guilty do you feel that she is being more noble and sacrificing than you would be for her if the situation was reversed?

- How embarrassed are you that she is being a better person than you would be if the roles were reversed?

- How angry do you feel that she is not being noble and sacrificing for you in your time of need?

- How angry are you that you would not treat her the way she is treating you if the roles were reversed?

- Do you hate her because she is indifferent and insensitive to your problem?

- Do you hate her because she was the one that jammed into your erection and started this whole mess?

- Do you feel like an old man without the sexual prowess you enjoyed with her before? Do you feel like a weakling, like you are defeated?

- Do you feel cheated that your sex life has been taken away from you?

- Are you disappointed in yourself causing this problem, or not doing something differently that might have prevented this from happening?

- Do you miss making love to her?

- Do you simply miss the close physical contact with her, holding her?

- Do you miss raunchy and wild sex with her?

- Is she the cause of many problems, because she feels guilty for injuring you and causing your PD? Have you forgiven her?

Why have you not told her these things? Perhaps because you are not sure of yourself. Perhaps because you are putting your needs ahead of hers. Perhaps you should be a man and make her a bigger part of your life. Talk to her.

Benefits of Communicating Like a Woman

Very simply, several direct and totally selfish benefits will come to a man who learns how to communicate better with his mate:

- It is the best and easiest way to express your commitment to her and to keep your marriage strong.

- It is the best way to keep her sexually interested in you, in spite of a malfunctioning penis – trust me.

- It is the best way to keep your own sanity; once you open up and feel the emotional freedom from your painful burden that this kind of discussion can bring, you will admit that these women know what they are doing.

Getting started

If you recognize the high importance of your wife's special needs to communicate, and how you previously have not fulfilled that need as well as you could have, now is the time to start communicating with her. Communicating is not just talking, although talking is the part of communication we tend to think about when the subject comes up. Listening is the other half of communication, and it is not as easy as you would think. Listening does not mean hearing; listening means paying attention to the speaker, following the discussion, paying attention to the flow of thought and giving consideration for what is being said. Good listening can sometimes be difficult.

It is not easy for men to open up at this level of honesty, vulnerability, and sincerity that women need. Young girls do this all the time in their social circles. Early in life they develop wonderful skills of compassionate and insightful communication between each other. Men seldom get into that level of communication. It is said that this social isolation in men contributes to their diminished happiness and early death; it is a significant reason, perhaps a primary reason, men die sooner than women.

119

To help you get started, please don't memorize this next paragraph, just read this as an idea of how to loosen yourself up a little. It takes a tough guy to feel exposed and still do it. Start out by saying something like this:

> "You know I don't like to talk about my feelings and things like that. I wasn't raised that way. It seems unnatural for me to discuss my feelings and my personal problems. I can't explain why, but maybe I feel like a sissy just thinking about talking about how I feel. But I know it is important for you and our marriage that I do this, so I am going to do this for us. It is especially difficult to talk about some of the things I am feeling since the Peyronie's disease started. I know I have not been good about expressing my feelings in the past, but I want you to know I am trying to change. I want to tell you what is going on inside my head and my heart. I want you to know exactly what has been bothering me so much lately and why I have been so difficult to be around lately. So here it is..."

Let it out. Open the flood gates and let it flow. Holding back would only hurt your effort, so be open and sincere. Enjoy the release.

If she knows as much as possible about this problem called Peyronie's disease, and how it has affected you as a person, she will be able to understand you better and deal with your situation in a way that might surprise you. You might very well find better understanding, and more tolerance of your lousy moods and bad behavior at times. You might find a better partner to share your troubles with, making a difficult time of life more tolerable for both of you.

The question is this: Can you be man enough to be more like a woman?

Communication with Your Children about PD

You must talk to your male children about PD. Like a lot of things associated with PD, this too is difficult but it absolutely must be done.

While it is imperative to discuss PD with your sons, it is a good idea for you or your wife to discuss PD in general terms with your daughter if she is married. You now have a compelling reason to have your daughter know about this problem from the standpoint of her knowing exactly how to avoid a PD problem for her partner. Consider how you could protect your daughter from a life of unhappiness and hardship by warning her about PD. A good father would do that for his daughter, no matter his personal discomfort. For these reasons, talk to all of your children, but most especially your son because of possible genetic predisposition considerations. There is no better day or time than right now.

It is cowardly and unfair to not warn your sons about the dangers of PD simply because you are embarrassed or uncomfortable. Do not delay. It is necessary to fess up to the situation and explain what you know so that your son might not make the same mistakes that you have made, and thus be spared what you are going through. It is far more important to put aside your discomfort and awkwardness for the welfare of your children.

For many, a discussion about PD with your sons is even more difficult than having a similar conversation with your wife. In modern culture it is still not customary for a man to reveal to his male offspring that he has a weakness anywhere, least of all in the area of sexual ability. Perhaps this gets back to the "old bull, young bull" relationship between father and son. A father often assumes the role of the strong one in the family, the tough one, the one who can take care of things. PD upsets all of that – a man is made to feel flawed in a most important and vital way, and no longer the "bull" that he once was. Even when strong father and son rivalry does not exist it can be difficult to reveal perceived weakness and limitation.

Different content levels

Not all PD discussions with your children should be the same. The actual content and frankness of your conversation about PD differ from situation to situation, primarily depending on the age and maturity of your children. The goal is to educate them honestly and fully about PD, with only specific information about your particular problem to serve as a general example (or maybe none). The information about your own PD situation should be as vague and protected, or as specific and detailed, as you think is beneficial for your children to learn; your penis and sex life should not necessarily be the focus of the discussion. The goal is to educate about PD, not embarrass yourself or your children. However, since sex talks are often mildly embarrassing at the start, your comfort or discomfort should not be an important consideration. The overriding motive should be to protect your children by presenting whatever level of information you believe is necessary for their PD education.

It might be of some small comfort to you to know that the older child will probably be more embarrassed than you are at the start of the conversation. Soon, after just a sentence of two, you will both become more relaxed. Make it easy on yourself and him by good strong initial eye contact to demonstrate that you are comfortable talking about this subject. It is also a good idea to make it a point to use the word "penis" right away, avoiding street terms.

Depending on the age of the child you are talking to, reviewing some of the anatomy and physiology on the **PDI** web site, or other medical web sites, would probably be a good idea. Perhaps jotting down a few pertinent facts and statistics might be interesting, too.

121

The important thing to emphasize is that the penis is made of delicate tissue that can sometimes be injured easily. The injury can be mild or severe, but is always difficult and slow to treat. Sometimes recovery is possible and sometimes it is not. Use the standard explanation of the piece of tape on the balloon to explain how the bend occurs (it's also on the **PDI** web site if you are not familiar with it). Emphasize that pain and distortion occur. If the child is very young, probably no mention needs to be made of impotence and loss of sexual activity. If it is a teenager that you are speaking to, then a phrase like, "… because of the scar the penis becomes bent and curved when erect. This can lead to the penis not working correctly," or "…and this extra scar tissue in the penis makes it curve when erect. The bend can make normal sexual activity difficult or impossible." Again, the content and level of explanation will depend on your audience.

This discussion is for your children's benefit. It should serve as a way to inform and educate to each child's level of curiosity and need to know about PD. The topic of discussion is PD, not "here's exactly how your lusty Mother turned into a wild woman one night and bent my penis." Do not embarrass your spouse or yourself mercilessly if it does not help your children. Little value is gained. However, let us assume that it was indeed you wife who injured your penis during intercourse. If appropriate for the older or married child, you can simply say that, "PD can sometimes be traced back to bending of the penis that accidentally happens during sexual activity." Further, you can protect the sexual details that describe how you developed your problem by telling your children you absolutely can not recall injuring yourself; you are one of those whose PD just developed without a reason you can recall. You can stonewall all of your personal details, if that is the way you want it.

Outline for Explaining PD to Your Child

Whether your son is in kindergarten or is a married man with children of his own, please read all the information in each of these three age groups because each expresses a slightly different idea that can be helpful no matter the age of your son.

Young Child (Potty Training Age to 10 Years of Age)

Think of this as an extension of all of the other training and instruction you have given your son for his protection. You have already discussed simply and directly how he should brush his teeth, wash his hands, not pick his nose in public, and comb his hair. These were all done in a minute or two with no huge fanfare or discomfort. This PD instruction should be the same.

1. **When**. Have the conversation at an appropriate time when the topic is natural. Start when you are in the bathroom together and perhaps you or he has just finished urinating. Start especially if you see him doing something that might injure his penis, or if he is running around the house without any clothes on. Look for the opportunity and it will occur.

122

2. **Dialogue example.** Speak in personal terms of "your penis," or "your private part," so there is no question that this applies to him, not "a penis" or "the penis."

Matter-of-factly state, "You know, your penis is made of really delicate tissue, and it can be hurt if you are not careful. You should be more careful when you are pulling your penis out of your pants. You should be more careful when you are playing outside so you do not hurt it. Your penis can be hurt very easily when it gets hard and big. (If you have never talked about erections, this might be a good time to answer his questions. Don't overload him with too much information if he does not ask or show that he specifically wants to know more.) Sometimes a boy can touch his penis when it is big and hard and it feels good. But if he bends it, or gets rough with it when it is big and hard, sometimes the hurt doesn't go away for a long time. So I want you to be more careful with yourself from now on. OK? You should be slower and more gentle when you pull yourself out when you go to the bathroom, especially if your penis is big and hard. OK? This is important so you do not hurt yourself. OK? Any questions?"

For additional ideas of how to instruct him, and things to talk about, to take better care of himself, go to Chapter 6, "Helpful Advice to Follow."

3. **Anatomy.** No special information is probably necessary. If you have a "family name" for the penis, "hot dog" or whatever, continue to use that familiar word with him – and "your penis" – so this discussion makes a lot of sense to him.

4. **Personal information about you.** None necessary.

5. **Follow up conversations.** As often as it seems appropriate. If you find him playing rough and carelessly the way youngsters do, you should remind him that he should be more careful, and why. If you find him masturbating, discuss it in the way your ethics and morals dictate. When you discuss masturbation in whatever way you think appropriate, you should repeat the idea of not being rough or bending the erect penis.

Older Child (From 7 to 18 Years of Age)

The most sad and tragic conversations I have with my PD audience are with scared 17-18 year-old boys who have PD and are too frightened to talk to their folks about it. They are so scared and embarrassed they do nothing more that read about it on the internet, and worry. They realize an important part of their lives is perhaps gone before it has even started. It is really sad.

Late last night I received an email from an 18 year-old boy who thinks he has PD. He used the word "suicide" three times, and begged for information to help him through his depression. I will call him, and arrange for professional help.

It is so important to inform your teenage son about everything you know concerning PD and its complications. I talk to too many young men who fell into a problem they did not know existed – had never heard of – simply out of ignorance. Like one young fellow told me, "I was just playing rough while it was hard. I would not have been doing that if I would have known this could happen." They are usually too exuberant in their frequent sexual activity at this young age and just do not know any better, until it is too late. Warn your son.

1. **When.** The sooner the better, probably today. He might be genetically predisposed, so you owe it to him. As a boy gets older he engages in heavier sports activity, the frequency of nocturnal erections increases, his sexual curiosity increases, his occasion for masturbation increases, and he is more at risk for PD. He is less likely to present a natural setting for this discussion, so just create the opportunity. While going somewhere in the car, or when you alone for an extended time to talk without interruption, is good enough.

2. **Dialogue example.** Speak in terms of "your penis" and not "a penis" or "the penis." Make it easy for him to relate to what you are saying to him. Use the words, "Peyronie's (pay-ro-neez) disease" often so it can sink into his memory.

   Matter-of-factly state, "You know, you are growing up and I see more and more you are behaving like an adult. I feel like I can talk to you as an equal. Because you are older, I want to tell you about some really important things you should know because you are becoming a man. This concerns your penis. You should not feel embarrassed or feel funny talking to me about these things because this is the way it is with men. If it's the truth and it's important, we should be able to just say what is on our minds without hesitation or embarrassment. I want you to know about some things that you have never even heard about before. I know you have not learned about this subject at school or when you talk to your buddies."

   "This is about a way that you can hurt yourself, your penis, today, that can stay with you forever. It is called Peyronie's disease. To explain how terrible it can be, if it is really a bad case it can even keep you from ever getting another erection for the rest of your life; it's like your penis is broke, and won't ever get hard again. It can maybe even keep you from ever becoming a father. I want to talk to you for a couple of minutes about Peyronie's disease. This is a really unusual problem that affects a man's

124

penis in a lot of different ways, and it is different for each person who gets it. Many things are unknown about this weird problem, but what is known is that Peyronie's disease can start sometimes after just a little injury to the penis that you might not even notice at the time. You do not have to get you penis slammed in a car door (ouch!) for Peyronie's disease to start. In some cases it seems to come out of no where, or for some men after a surgical procedure to the penis, and even after taking certain kinds of drugs. Some people are more prone to get Peyronie's disease than others; some men are able to receive a lot of injury to the penis and nothing ever happens, and for other men it just starts after a little thing that is so minor that it is hardly remembered. There is no way to know if you or I are likely to get this problem so you just have to be careful and not take any chances with yourself. OK?"

"If you get Peyronie's disease it can be very painful every time you get an erection, although sometimes it is just minor pain. And the bend that develops can be small or really huge, like a corkscrew; can you imagine that? Wow, that would be terrible. If your penis is bent like that, besides being painful, it sometimes is so bad that you cannot even get an erection and that would not be good either. You know that you need to have an erection to become a father, right? OK?"

"I want you to be safe and healthy, and I want you to not have any problems like Peyronie's disease. So I want you to think about being more careful with yourself when you go to the bathroom to urinate. I read that a penis is most likely to get injured and start a case of Peyronie's disease when it is erect. That is just because of the way it is built with layers of tissue that can become separated if it is bent suddenly. So when you have an erection it is very important that you do not get rough with it or have any goofy accidents with it. OK? Do you have any questions at all? OK? Good."

For additional ideas of how to instruct him, and things to talk about, to take better care of himself, go to Chapter 6, "Helpful Advice to Follow."

3. **Anatomy**. It is probably a good idea to be more technical and authoritative by using a few anatomical terms just to show that you know what you are talking about (especially if he is a teenager). Look up the words, "corpora," "tunica," and "plaque" on the **PDI** web site. Use them, and explain them, matter-of-factly. It would go something like this, "Inside the penis is a very thin tissue layer called the 'tunica albuginea' or just 'tunica' that is like a protective layer. It is strong but delicate, so it can get injured easily.

"This tunica covers the main tissue of the penis on the inside that is called the 'corpora'. The tunica is like the skin on a hot dog, and the meat of the hot dog is like the corpora, and all of this is under the skin of your penis."

"This corpora is different from any other tissue in the body because it swells up and holds blood sometimes; this is how an erection happens. The tunica that covers the corpora does not have a good blood supply, so any injury there heals slowly. The injury causes a scar inside that is called a 'plaque'. When a plaque forms it can prevent the corpora from swelling up normally during an erection. It works this way: The plaque is like a piece of tape. The corpora is like a long balloon. If the balloon is not blown up with air it is small and limp. When the balloon is blown up with air it gets big and firm. The air is like blood that goes into the corpora. Got it? OK. If you put a piece of tape on a balloon and then blow it up, the balloon will not inflate correctly, and it will be bent. If that happens to the penis it is called Peyronie's disease. It hurts, it can bend the penis into weird shapes and it can prevent the penis from working correctly. Any questions? Everything OK? Good."

Lead him to the **PDI** web site if he has more questions.

It might be a good idea to review the **PDI** web site about erections before you talk to him.

4. **Personal information about you.** It might not be necessary if he is still young, but if you feel that it would be helpful to mention that you have PD, by all means give him the information you feel is important. For more ideas of what to tell him about your problem, refer to the section that follows.

5. **Follow up conversations.** When appropriate. If you find a natural time to bring it up again, you only need to remind him to be careful. If you are having some other conversation with him about sex, try to work PD into that conversation. If you find him masturbating, you should handle it in the way that your ethics and morals dictate. In addition, you should at that time repeat the idea of not being rough or bending the erect penis.

Suggest that he checks out some of the pages of the **PDI** web site to help him understand this problem better.

Adult Son (16 Years of Age and Up)

1. **When.** Personally, I would take it as a great personal failure on my part if I did not warn my son about PD, and he developed it while I was making excuses why I should wait a little longer to have that talk. Make time to have a good heart to heart discussion with your grown son to tell him what you know about PD; the sooner the better.

2. **Dialogue example.** Here is how I laid out the Peyronie's disease facts for my two adult sons a few years back. I felt the need to stress the possibility that they could be genetically predisposed to PD, and made sure they knew how nasty my case was, and how difficult it was to deal with emotionally for a while. I urged that they act on what I was telling them about being very careful with their personal behavior. I stressed how disruptive and unsettling this was for a while to my relation with their mother, my wife. I made sure that each understood that PD is perhaps the largest physical problem and personal tragedy that has ever entered my life.

Matter-of-factly state, "I want to talk to you about something that is really important. The first thing I want you to know is that I have a non-fatal, a non-life threatening, disease of the reproductive system called Peyronie's disease. This isn't going to kill me, OK? But it is a nasty health problem, understand? It is a terrible problem of fibrous tissue developing in the internal tissue of the penis. This fibrous tissue is called a plaque or scar. It prevents the penis from filling out straight when it is erect. What I am telling you right now is not necessarily for you to know about my problem in particular, but for you to be informed about Peyronie's disease so that you do not develop it yourself. Peyronie's disease has some very strong evidence for genetic predisposition, so it is certainly possible you could develop it. Believe me, I would not wish this problem on my worst enemy. Men have committed suicide over this problem. Besides the pain, and the reduction of sexual function, (yes, your mother and I are still alive,) my penis developed one terribly nasty double bend that was really difficult to deal with from an emotional standpoint. After using a lot of Alternative Medicine treatments I am back to normal. I worked hard to help myself, and I got well; some men never do. I want you to know as much about this as you can, so you can avoid this problem. I will give you the address of a web site to get more information. It has pictures, diagrams and will answer all of your questions about every aspect of Peyronie's disease. OK? Will you do that? Good."

3. **Anatomy**. Read the discussion that is given for the previous age group.

4. **Personal information about you.** That is entirely up to you. Personally, I wanted to make this very real for my two sons, so I gave a lot more physical details to my sons than I have indicated in the above sample dialogue. I wanted to make sure they took this as seriously as possible. I wanted to jolt them with some hard facts and scary ideas of how nasty this problem can be, and I did.

However, if you do not want to reveal the embarrassing truth of how you got your PD one wild and crazy night with their mother, then you can always say simply that you have no idea how your PD developed. You can explain that you are in that 50% group in which PD seems to come out of nowhere. No need to embarrass yourself or your wife – or your son, for that matter.

5. **Follow up conversations.** Over the next few months I asked each boy if he had spent much time on the **PDI** web site. I asked if there were any questions or problems in understanding any section. It was simply my instinct that I am still their father, and even though they are both bigger than I am, it is still my responsibility and privilege to take care of them in whatever way that I can.

Communication with Parents If You Are Under 21 Years Old

The average age for onset of PD is about 50-55 years of age. PD can begin as late as into the 80s, and at the other end of the age spectrum, it can start in the mid-to-latter teen years. Since the incidence of PD increases with age, with the peak age of onset somewhere around 53 years, it would be logical that the occurrence of teen PD is rather low compared to older age brackets. However, an accurate estimate of the number of teenagers with PD is more difficult to make than in the general population because of the additional cultural, emotional and social issues related to youth.

Despite a relatively low occurrence of PD in the youthful population, a serious aspect of teen PD makes it extremely important to address. The gravity of PD in these teen cases is they are barely more than boys who encounter such a crushing physical and emotional trauma in their lives, totally unprepared. Many young men may simply lack the many resources needed to deal effectively with such a sobering and heavy burden. At this young age they lack the emotional maturity to handle the plight alone, and in their shock and confusion are often inclined to isolate themselves from parents and professional help due to embarrassment about sexual matters. Perhaps the most compelling concern for this age group arises from a teen's anger and depression evolving into a suicidal response, after he realizes PD is a lifelong tragedy that has stopped his sexual life before it has begun.

Based on the frequency of contact by these teens who clandestinely call or email **PDI** for an opinion about a strange curvature suggestive of PD, it appears the number of teens who have PD is grossly underestimated.

Undiagnosed Problem

Most teens who contact **PDI** for advice have not been medically examined for their suspected PD problem. Often the problem has continued for many months prior to the time **PDI** is contacted.

From data collected by **PDI** over a two-year period these are the primary situations during which they suspect their PD started:

1. Sexual intercourse without parents' knowledge
2. Masturbation, usually of a very rough and ritualistic nature
3. Insertion of "things" into the urethra, the opening at the tip of the penis
4. Homosexual intercourse
5. During a simultaneous violent epileptic seizure and nocturnal erection

Because these young men often withhold this information from all adults, their problem is unexamined, undiagnosed, and untreated. As a group these are bright and articulate young men who have researched their symptoms on the Internet, in an effort to determine the nature of their problem. They display an above average layperson's understanding of PD. But even with a good technical understanding of the PD problem, they are still unsure the PD diagnosis applies to them. Most of the time, from the experience of **PDI**, these young men are overreacting and do not have PD.

However, no one will ever know if a teenager's problem is actually PD until it is medically diagnosed. This is the purpose of this particular discussion.

Several Possible Options

When a young man notices a bump, lump or bend in his penis that was not present previously, only a few possibilities can usually be considered until a professional examination establishes a definitive diagnosis. Until that time, there are several concerns in these cases:

1. **If the condition is not PD** – There are two different extremes to explain the curved penis that concerns the teen:

   A. **It is just a slight normal variation** in which the penis is normally not straight. Not all people are perfectly even or symmetrical in every part of the body. The face is often not balanced or even, the two hands and feet are not always exactly alike, a woman's breasts are often of uneven size and shape, and so the penis – being made of two separate corpora or cylindrical bodies – can also be of different size causing a normal bend or curve. A teen without full medical background does not possess sufficient knowledge to make an accurate diagnosis of PD, yet his concern causes him to focus on the presence of a normally curved penis.

   B. **It is some other health problem, not PD**. While even more rare than PD, other problems with the urethra or other penile tissue can occur that should receive medical attention. In these situations delay of examination, diagnosis and treatment is not in the best interest of the young man.

2. **If the condition actually is PD** – When all necessary symptoms are present, medical examination is still needed to make an accurate diagnosis of PD. Everything that must be done to restore life back to order begins with a formal diagnosis of PD; a teenager cannot do that on his own, no one can without medical attention. No benefit, real or imagined, can come from delay of knowing exactly the nature of the problem. The continual stress and worry that arises from not knowing the exact nature of your problem is much greater than confronting the problem directly.

In either case, whether you have PD or not, prompt action and learning the truth are always preferable to not knowing the exact nature of a health problem. Anyone with a potential medical problem needs to receive correct care promptly. To delay, allowing an undiagnosed condition to worsen, is a huge mistake.

Reluctance to Talk to Parents

Teens are often uncommunicative to their parents for a variety of social, developmental and psychological reasons. From ongoing experience with young men who contact **PDI** for advice and opinions, it is apparent that many teenagers go to great lengths and endure significant hardships to keep their suspected PD problem a secret from their parents.

I have communicated with men in their early 20s who have kept knowledge of their suspected PD from their parents for many years. The reluctance that causes them to keep their problem to themselves sometimes centers on the concern for over-reaction and fear of punishment from one or both parents. It is not the PD that prevents the teen from talking to his parents. The refusal to talk to his parents typically comes from fear of how the parent will respond to the type of sexual activity, or the person, that was involved when he thinks he injured himself. His dread is over his parent's response to the start of the problem and not the problem itself. Our contact with these teens is very brief, and seldom seems to lead to the teen's parents ever being informed. No opportunity for follow-up contact is ever provided.

Necessity to Inform a Parent

If you are a teenage male, a legal minor, it is necessary for certain technical medicolegal steps to occur before examination and treatment can be given to you. State laws differ throughout the country in this regard, but young women are generally more protected in this area than young men. Specific information in regard to your state should be determined before you proceed. Authorization by a responsible adult, who has a recognized family relationship to you, must be given to medical personnel in order for care to be provided. Standard release documents must be signed, and proof of financial responsibility for care must be provided. In other words, a parent or other responsible authorized relative must come forward to take full responsibility for your care. Without parental knowledge and cooperation, medical care is essentially unavailable in some states and in certain situations.

A teen who isolates himself from his parents because of PD can make his situation worse by the lack of emotional and financial support, as well as the need for a wide range of advice and decisions that will be made over time.

As an option, you should find a trusted adult who you can go to for help about approaching your parents. This can be an older brother, an uncle, a teacher from school, or someone from your church. This person can help you speak to your parents about your problem.

If Parental Problems Prevent You from Getting Help

Every family has problems, and some are extremely bad. A teen might be living in a hostile and deprived environment that creates a poor family relationship. If a teen with suspected PD finds himself in that kind of situation in which turning to his parents for help with a problem like PD is a dangerous course of action, or they are simply unavailable to him for a variety of reasons, then he must take action in another direction.

If a teen cannot talk to his parents about his PD problem, then he must talk to an adult who can help – an older brother, an uncle, an adult who is trusted and available for assistance, the school nurse who can direct him to other social agencies, or a clinic where help is available for people who cannot pay.

How to Talk to Your Parents about Your Problem

There are parents who are good, and others who are not.

If you have a good relationship with your folks, and they are good to deal with, then go to them and tell them what you have found. Be open and honest. Ask for help and cooperate with them in whatever way you are asked.

If your folks are not around to help you, or if you have a bad and hostile relationship with your folks, and you are worried a huge blowup could happen if they learned you have a problem with your penis, then you must take action to protect yourself and still get some help. If you do not trust how one or both of your parents might respond to this information, you should probably limit what you tell them so that you do not place yourself in danger. If you know you cannot or should not talk to your parents based on past reactions from them, there are ways you can use to prevent or limit the reaction you fear from them.

First, remember that you will be in total control of all information that could be embarrassing, damaging to your relationship with your parents, or harmful to you. While it is always better to provide full and accurate information about any health problem, how you think your PD started is really unimportant from the standpoint of medical care. What you were doing, who was with you, and how you assume the problem started can almost be seen as rather unimportant medically.

Any medical doctor who takes your history knows that in about 50% of the cases of PD no recollection of a specific injury or event that actually started the problem will ever be made. These cases just seem to develop on their own, without any trauma at all. If it makes you feel more comfortable, and allows you to come forward to get help, then that is how you present your problem. Your story can be that there was no injury or specific event, and no one can argue that you are not correct. However, all other information about your penis that you give to your doctor must be true and accurate.

Therefore, embarrassment about background details and fear of parental punishment should be unnecessary. While total honesty is always the best policy, if you feel the need to protect yourself from an abusive or uncaring family situation you should do so. In this way, you protect yourself from parental reprisal and still get the care you need.

Not Important How You Think You Got Your PD

Even if you think you are absolutely positive you know how your PD started, in actual fact you might be wrong. Do not place yourself in jeopardy with your parents if you fear their reaction, and do not avoid medical care out of embarrassment over how you assume your PD started, because you might be incorrect. Since no one will ever actually know – not even you – and no huge benefit comes from knowing how it started, do not allow how your problem started, to be the barrier that keeps you from being helped.

If you think your problem started while having sex during a drunken or drug- induced episode, it is essentially unimportant to the doctor who would be examining or treating you. What is far more important to your doctor is the speed of progression of your problem, the amount of pain you are having, how it affects your daily life, and so on. If you had sex with Tina or Tim is not important to your doctor; only your current and future health matters. If you hurt yourself in some strange act of masturbation involving a watermelon, that fact is not as important as your recovery. Therefore, you can keep this kind of information to yourself.

What to Say to Your Parents If You Feel Unsafe

You are going to your parents to ask for help. Your explanation should serve as a way to inform and educate your parents about PD, and how it relates to you. The topic of discussion is PD and what to do to get help, not "here's what I think I did to injure my penis." There is no point in speculating about something that you cannot know for sure, that might unnecessarily put you at odds with your folks. Little to no value is gained if you guess how your PD started. The safest and best approach is to put yourself in the group of 50% of men whose PD just comes out of nowhere like a mystery, because it could actually be the truth.

Please do not try to memorize any of this. Use it only as an example of how to handle this discussion with your folks.

1. **When.** If possible, talk to one or both of your parents today. Without an easy or natural way to bring it up, make the time and just do it.

2. **Dialogue example.** Don't talk like a street person, or talk dirty to your parents, especially if your mother is part of this discussion. Don't say "cock," "dick," or whatever, and expect to be treated in a way that you want to be treated. If you speak like a mature adult, you are more likely to be treated like a mature adult. Use terms like "my penis is bent," "my private part is getting sore," or "it hurts down there." You probably do not speak to your friends in those terms, but for the purpose of this talk with your parents you should show respect and not add stress to the relations between you and them.

   Once you get going you will feel less embarrassed; it will get easier.

   Matter-of-factly state, "Mom, Dad, I have a problem I have to talk to you about. About a few weeks/months ago I found a little bump on my penis when I was in the bathroom. It really scared me. I looked up information on the Internet and I think it is a problem called Peyronie's disease. They call it some kind of mystery disease because so little is known about it, and in about half of the cases no cause is ever found – it just starts out of nowhere.

   "I have no idea how it started, but that is part of this condition; like I said, about half of the people with it don't have any injury or anything that explains how it stated. Sometimes it runs in families, like diabetes or high blood pressure. Do you know of any men in our family who have Peyronie's disease? Well, anyway, getting back to what is happening to me down there ..."

   Explain your problem with PD to the best of your ability, and still be comfortable and unembarrassed. Explain what you know about Peyronie's disease to help them understand what you know.

Answer their questions as best you can. Invite them to the **PDI** web site to learn more about it for themselves if they want to know more.

Be prepared that they will be upset, shocked and not understand at first. Give them time to absorb the fact that you have a health problem that they have never heard about. Anyone would be initially confused and upset. Try not to respond to any anger or frustration from them with a similar response. Stay calm and explain yourself.

3. **Anatomy** No special information is probably necessary. You can use terms like "tunica" and "corpora" and "plaque" to help you explain the problem if you want.

4. **Personal information about you.** Explain what your problem is in a way that is not embarrassing to you. Both of your parents know about erections. If you are not comfortable saying "erection" in front of your parents, then just say "when it gets hard." You might be surprised to know that maybe your parents are just as uneasy talking about sex with you, as you are with them. It's a crazy thing in our culture, but it's true. Speak as generally as you can while still explaining your problem.

5. **Follow up conversations.** Leave it up to them to ask how you are doing. If they do not ask for whatever reason – it just might be out of embarrassment, or to give you some privacy – then just let it go. If they ask, answer in a comfortable way.

Good luck to you getting help and discussing your problem with your parents.

Chapter 10 – Dangers that Lurk Around the Corner

Ω - **To live a better life, be happier and healthier in spite of your PD, and increase your chance of successfully treating it …**

… you must not injure your penis or aggravate your PD further. You must be aware that certain things that you have always done, or even new things that you are tempted to do, might not be good for your PD. It is necessary to think about how your PD might be affected by many common and simple things around you that pose a danger to your recovery from PD. One of the reasons you might not be thinking in this way is that no one has ever told you about the things in this chapter. Read on, and learn.

With PD, the World Changes

Your mental attitude and appreciation of life have changed in some ways since you developed PD. These mental and emotional shifts probably have to do with what you think about yourself and your life now, compared to the way things used to be. You have probably noticed changes of an emotional nature within yourself. This response could be due to reduced or absent sexual activity, or perhaps in dreaded anticipation of future surgery, impotency or divorce. Most likely little else in your life has changed, with other external daily activities and behaviors continuing as before the presence of Peyronie's disease.

It is safe to assume you have not made any changes in your life in response to PD, except those that have been forced upon you by your circumstances. *Yet, there probably should be more deliberate change in your life than what you have already undertaken.* These changes should occur in response to what is good and what is bad for your PD. Once your eyes have been opened to the consequences of some of your actions, through this book and your expanded awareness, it should be a straightforward decision to alter your activities and choices in consideration of your personal situation.

Decisions Have Consequences

The idea that there are things around you – what you do, what and how you eat, what you wear, what happens to you – that should possibly be avoided or limited because they pose a real or potential danger to your PD, is new even to men who have had the problem for many years. It is the intent of this chapter to explain some of these situations to you, so that you can avoid further potential injury to the penis.

From the experience gained over the years in talking to men who have PD, I have come to learn that not one in a thousand men really understands his problem. Those few who have some understanding of the disease process have all been self-educated about PD. Some could even be considered experts in their own limited way. Those who come to know about PD have all done so out of frustration and self-determination. I have never communicated with anyone who felt that his medical doctor did more than just superficially explain PD. Their doctor never suggested certain "do's and don'ts" involved with PD; all have felt they had to figure certain things out for themselves, primarily based on common sense. No one has ever said that he had been educated about what to avoid or limit because of this problem with his penis. All were surprised by the information they were given by **PDI** about things to avoid or do differently because of the PD.

What You Do Not Know, and Do Not Do, Can Hurt You

Things that were unimportant before developing PD could be of considerable concern to you since you are now more vulnerable to additional penile injury. It is necessary to reconsider many small issues that previously were unimportant and inconsequential before.

Not understanding your problem is an extremely dangerous situation to be in. This danger is listed first because misunderstanding your problem is probably the greatest threat to your eventual recovery. You can't make good choices for yourself if you don't understand the problem, and you are far more likely to make bad choice for the same reason.

• Little to No Information Is Given to the PD Patient

In a climate in which not much good information is available about PD, much potential damage and difficulties can arise. Without learning about PD from your doctor during a routine examination, or in the written word that comes from books or the Internet, the sense of abandonment and confusion grows. PD has often been called the "orphan disease" because no one seems to care much about it or those who have it – except as a surgical opportunity. Over and over I learn that the average man stops going to his doctor for his PD because the atmosphere is one of disinterest. Questions and problems are not addressed, hurry in and hurry out, and limited time and opportunity is given for discussion. This is not a good atmosphere in which to receive information or instruction; no wonder so many men are totally in the dark about their problem, or at least very confused.

Recently I received an email from a man who wrote, *"I went to my family doctor about the lump on the side of my penis because it seemed to be causing an abrupt bend to the right. He said I should do nothing, because the problem with my penis would leave me just as quickly as it started. My doctor said that even vitamin E was a waste of time. That was over four years ago, and I am still waiting for it to leave. During that time my problem has gotten worse, my wife has left me, I do not even think about dating. I am so angry at the world and depressed I sometimes think about suicide.*" Following the advice that he was given was not only harmful to his potential recovery, it could be fatal if it leads further into his depths of emotional despair.

• *Vitamin E, and All the Others*

This discussion is rather long because vitamin E is one of the most common and basic forms of PD treatment that is undertaken. Most of the things said about the use, or misuse, of vitamin E could also be said of all other members of the Alternative Medicine group of therapies. Nutrition is a much misunderstood subject, not only by the average layperson but also by the average physician who has essentially no formal training in the area of human nutrition.

Many men with PD, based on my conversations, are simply told by their medical doctors to "take some vitamin E." Little information is given about dosage, when or how to take the supplements, or for what duration of time. Nothing is ever said about the quality of vitamin E supplementation, nor is a patient advised about the different physiologic and therapeutic benefits of natural organic vitamin E over the synthetic varieties. It is a mistaken belief of the average medical practitioner that a synthetic vitamin E is as good as a naturally occurring product. MDs think this way primarily because they are accustomed to prescribing chemically manufactured or artificial chemicals all the time. Therefore, they see no problem in prescribing a synthetic vitamin. Patients are left to purchase their vitamin E without adequate explanation about the various types of vitamin E. Believing the natural and synthetic have the same benefit, they usually buy the cheapest (and most inferior) vitamin E product they can find. No wonder so little success with vitamin E is reported under these circumstances. Valuable time, money, and opportunity for healing are wasted simply because the average doctor does not know any better and does not inform his patients correctly in this most important area of therapy.

Further danger is encountered when people with only sketchy information and limited experience are asked about specific forms of PD therapy. They will often answer in an authoritative manner, giving incorrect or incomplete information, or they will state their opinion as though it was fact. Even a perfectly good PD therapy like vitamin E can be bad-mouthed when someone, who used it incorrectly, gives his opinion of it. Here is a typical question from a man who recently joined an Internet chat room group devoted to Peyronie's disease, taken from a recent email message to the group, *"Have any of you taken Vitamin E, and does it make any difference in your opinion?"* This is a great question; it is usually presented to the wrong people, for the most part.

The great majority of men in these Peyronie's discussion groups are quick to answer a wide variety of technical and medical questions. They base their answers on their own bad experiences with all the therapies they have tried –

that is why they are still there as Peyronie's sufferers. For anyone who asks they will list all of the therapies they have tried, and conclude with an authoritative sounding opinion that "no treatment works for PD" simply because it did not work for them. What is difficult to learn from them, however, is exactly how they used the therapy. I have rarely, if ever, found a discussion in which adequate details of treatment were given. Most reports from men in the discussion groups simply state something like, "I tired it, and it didn't work." That's not only unhelpful, it could lead to the wrong impression of a perfectly good therapy that could have been performed incorrectly or too briefly, or with bargain-basement products that were doomed to fail due to low quality.

While there are always exceptions, such as well-versed and intelligent discussion group contributors, they are in the minority. For the person asking very sincere and probing questions, there is real risk in having absolutely no way of knowing the quality of the answer or the depth of knowledge and understanding on which it is based. None of these men explain how they used the vitamin E, the brand of vitamin E used, how long they took it, or how faithful they were to their plan, etc. Most replies will be along the lines of, "I tried vitamin E and all I can tell you is that it didn't make a bit of difference to me." This is the kind of question and answer format that fills thousands of pages of PD chat room conversations. The fellow who gave that answer could have purchased his vitamin E from Wal-Mart and taken 10 capsules over a one month period of time. The reader does not know this, nor does he appreciate that the information is inherently invalid. The danger is that people who do not know any better will take the word of a more experienced man as the absolute truth in all of these areas. The newcomer's future course of action will be influenced by people who might not have done anything correctly during their own care, and now offer opinions and direct others how to manage their treatment. This is a problem that I see over and over again in all of the chat rooms that I monitor. I am concerned that it is often a case of the blind leading others into the darkness, and no good comes of it.

The reader is left to conclude that a particular therapy is ineffective because that is the way the answer is presented. The thoughtful reader should know that it is also possible that the therapy is actually effective in a fair number of cases, but it was not used properly in the case being reported. This concept – that vitamin E is good, but perhaps the man with the bad experience with vitamin E might just have done it incorrectly in one way or another – is never mentioned. In the atmosphere of a PD discussion group, this kind of reply would cause cruel personal attacks and verbal warfare that would continue for days, amongst the irritable and angry men who spend their time there. No, what happens is that a biased opinion is presented as fact, it is never questioned by the group, and it passes as the truth for the men who are new to PD. Thus, misinformation continues to spread and sadly nothing changes much in the world of PD.

For an in-depth explanation of the types, use, and results of correct vitamin E therapy, please visit the **PDI** web site at www.peyronies-disease-help.com and click on the "Therapy Options" tab where you will then find a discussion of "Vitamin E & C."

• *Wait-and-See Strategy*

One of the most dangerous and damaging suggestions that men receive from their doctor when they are first told they have PD, is to basically do nothing for the first year or two. This popular approach of merely observing a case of PD for a while is used because in about 50% of cases the scar and curvature might spontaneously disappear without any care being provided. This is the famous "wait-and-see approach" to treating PD.

The medical thinking is this: "In half of cases the PD goes away on its own, so there is no point in doing anything. If it doesn't go away, we can always operate." For the half of the PD cases that do not go away, the scar and problem either stay the same or get a lot worse. If the PD results in an "acceptable" level of pain, an "acceptable" degree of penile distortion, or an "acceptable" level of sexual impairment, the outcome of PD is said to be "acceptable" or "satisfactory" and the MD who prescribed this wait-and-see strategy thinks this approach was successful for that individual. For this reason, the doctor will likely suggest the wait-and-see strategy for the next case of PD he sees. The MD is happy with the "acceptable" outcome of this non-care, even though his patient has filed for divorce and is thinking of suicide.

This wait-and-see approach for the first year is based on the doctor's sincere hope that the scar will eventually resolve into an "acceptable" penile problem. Please re-read that last part of the sentence: "…the doctor's sincere hope that the scar will eventually resolve into an 'acceptable' penile problem."

At the beginning of care, when the wait-and-see approach is first offered as a valid way of handling this problem, the doctor has already given up on the patient actually getting well, and will be pleased if the patient has an "acceptable" level of pain, curvature, and loss of sexual function. It should be of interest to any patient to know that his problem is not being treated to be cured or actively helped. It should be of interest to any PD patient to know that his case is being put on hold for a year to see if he becomes an "acceptable" penile freak. So if the scar, pain and resultant bend develop within a predetermined "acceptable" level, then the doctor's opinion will be that everything worked out pretty well – even if the patient doesn't think so.

Can you believe that this is the thinking behind the wait-and-see strategy. And what if your PD results in an "unacceptable" level of scar formation, pain, and resultant bend? Oh, surgery can be done! Just a little snip, snip here and there, and you will be as good as you can be. Men hearing their doctor's explanation that surgery is the back-up treatment of choice want to believe that it will get them back to normal, and don't really find out how often the results are a failure or worse.

For more discussion of PD surgery, refer to http://peyronies-disease-help.com/peyronies-disease-surgery.html

- *Just What Is a "Satisfactory" or "Acceptable" Outcome?*

You should find out early in your care if it is your doctor's opinion that a 5-10-20° bend in your penis is a "satisfactory" outcome in his or her estimation. You should find out early in your care if it is your doctor's opinion that it is not worth the trouble of perhaps taking some enzymes and a few other supplements during this first year to see if you can do something to help yourself out a little. You should find out if it is your doctor's opinion that not being able to have intercourse normally – as you have done previously – for the rest of your life is a "satisfactory" outcome, and is not worth the trouble of perhaps doing some exercises and using DMSO with copper and vitamin E. You should find out early if it is your doctor's opinion that a dull ache and throb (maybe even a sharp pain) in your private parts every time you happen to get an erection is a "satisfactory" outcome, and is not worth the effort of perhaps following a nutritional program of MSM, vitamins E and C, Japanese herbs and maybe some carnitine.

Perhaps a good question to ask your doctor is this one:

"Which of these two options would you suggest is the best treatment for me to take:

1. Surgery, with a 40-50% failure rate (always resulting in loss of about 1-2 inches of penis length, and possible impotency).

2. Use of Alternative Medicine therapy that has few, if any known side-effects, but has not yet been proven to cure PD."

It might be interesting to learn what your doctor thinks is a reasonable course of treatment for you. Carefully read those medical web sites that discuss PD treatment options. You will find how common is the opinion that so long as the penis is not terribly distorted and extremely painful, then everything is "acceptable."

If you have PD, you should know that the medical profession has a very low standard by which to judge what an "acceptable" level of pain and distortion is for YOUR penis, and what is an "acceptable" level of sexual impairment in YOUR bedroom. Using their own standards by which to judge the health and well-being of YOUR penis, the medical profession has determined that this wait-and-see treatment approach makes sense

140

to them. But, _does it make sense to YOU_? At the beginning of your PD treatment you should know if your doctor is willing to take a chance like this with YOUR penis, when there are many reasonable conservative treatment options – even if they are currently unproven. PDI thinks this wait-and-see approach is a poor gamble and a bad strategy.

The watch-wait-and-do-nothing strategy for PD must sound good only to the surgeon. To **PDI** it sounds like playing Russian Roulette with very bad odds. At least in Russian Roulette only one bullet is in a six-cylinder gun; that's a one out of six chance of losing. In the wait-and-see approach, half of the cases clear up spontaneously; that's a one out of two chance of losing. Or to put it another way, that's like playing Russian Roulette with three bullets in a six-cylinder gun. No thanks.

Most would agree that it is better to do all that you can for your PD, as soon as you can, using as many of the safe and scientifically grounded options that are known to have some limited success in helping the PD scar heal. If after following an aggressive alternative medical program, such as is presented on the **PDI** web site, a man gains less than complete repair and healing – as can happen – then surgery can still be used.

You are taking a chance that the currently unproven alternative therapies **PDI** advocates might not work for you, but the down-side risk is minimal for the most part. We leave it to the reader to decide which is the greater risk: ignoring the problem, or exploring an uncharted treatment area. For further discussion, please visit the **PDI** web site at www.peyronies-disease-help.com

Vulnerable Times When You Have PD

Both early and late stages of PD are times of personal danger because of the great vulnerability that is at play with this emotionally charged problem.

In the early stage of the disease, when you first learn that you have PD, you are likely to be too confused and scared to think straight. You are given a diagnosis that you have never heard of before, and you aren't even sure how to pronounce it, let alone spell it. You don't want to believe what you are hearing. It is difficult to understand the strange new terms and concepts. If you are lucky, you get too much information that comes too fast and most of it is simply not absorbed. If you are not lucky, as happens to the vast majority of men, you get little information and are left to figure things out for yourself.

Because no layperson can be sufficiently knowledgeable about this strange mystery disease that is dumped in his lap, it is impossible to know how to handle the situation early in care. The layperson is caught off guard by a problem he never heard of before. Initially he does not know enough about his problem to identify good and bad information. He can neither ask intelligent questions, nor comprehend initially how little sense the wait-and-see approach makes.

In the later stage of the disease there are new levels of vulnerability and danger that develop over time.

After a year or so of enduring PD most men are tired of doing nothing, desperate to do something to save a foundering marriage and regain some degree of self-esteem. Life is no longer good. Much of the prior marital stability is either gone or is seriously eroded. This pressure and sense of personal distraction do not make for positive or levelheaded decision making. Some marriages get stronger while enduring the ravages of PD, but these are the exception.

If a man is faithfully following his doctor's advice about vitamin E, he surely does not know that he is using only a small fraction of the wide group of conservative Alternative Medicine therapies that are available to him. He assumes that his doctor has done all of the homework for him, and is actually helping him in whatever way is available. Usually, this is not true.

The medical patient with PD thinks that the only acceptable therapy plan is to first do nothing for a while. Next, verapamil cream or verapamil injections are tried. After that does not work, then in desperation "some vitamin E" is used, but the doctor is not too excited about it because in his or her limited experience and knowledge, vitamin E never seems to help any patient. After that, if things get really bad for the poor guy with PD, then the last available option is to go visit the surgeon.

Little does the man, going the medical route of treatment, know his doctor is just hoping that the PD will result in an "acceptable" level of scar formation, pain, distortion, only "limited" erectile dysfunction, and "acceptable" loss of sexual ability. And little does he know the care he is being given is much less than the wide variety of therapies available to him. He is not aware that he and his problem are being – without a better way to say it – ignored. His options have not been explored or discussed with him, and he is not doing all that he could do to help himself.

In this later stage of PD, when surgery is mentioned perhaps for the second or third time by the treating doctor, first a sense of panic sets in, usually followed by rejection of the therapy that is called "the only real cure." At this point a man will start to look for treatment options on his own.

Going to the Internet, he finds little solid information about getting better. Most of what he reads is a discussion of what does not work, and the final solution of surgery. He learns that the reason for his doctor's indifference to this problem is because everything about PD is unknown and unproven, and each case is unchartered territory.

After being on the Internet for a while, he is filled with hopelessness and frustration. The medical profession that does miraculous things for all of the other health problems in the world just doesn't know much about PD. He sees this statement over and over again, but it does not make sense that limbs can be re-attached and cancer can be cured, but no one knows much about PD. Ah, how sad it is to be the neglected orphan of the medical world!

Pessimism and indecision abound from all sources of information. Negativity and reports of poor response come not only from the professional and research groups, but also from the layman's discussion groups. Of course, the Internet discussion groups only repeat the doom and gloom opinion of their medical physicians, and repeat their own bad experiences from using small doses of cheap synthetic vitamin E, or topical Verapamil. So at this time the average guy with PD is not sure how far his problem will advance, if his penis will turn into a corkscrew, or leave him totally impotent. He is experiencing major unhappiness and insecurity at home. His wife or girlfriend is talking about leaving him, and he is unsure of this ability to ever attract or keep another mate. He knows he is losing an important part of life, he is losing his maleness, and he does not know what to do about any of it. He begins to think dark thoughts, if you know what I mean.

This is another dangerous time for the man with PD. If this describes a little of what is happening to you, please go to the **PDI** web site and get some information about the wide variety of Alternative Medicine treatment options – over a dozen of them – and get yourself involved in building up your health and vitality so you can do the best job possible of reversing your own PD. Self-repair is done in over half of the cases, why not you?

Pornography and Penis Enlargement Get in the Way of PD Treatment

Many web sites that appear during an Internet search about PD are just pornography and/or penis enlargement sites. Anyone who has spent even a short time on the Internet looking for PD information has run into a wide variety of them. These web sites have been programmed to pop up when any request is made for information about PD. It doesn't mean they actually have anything to do with PD; they just come up with the rest of the PD information. This is a danger to your PD only because it is a distraction of time, money, and energy that should be placed in genuinely productive areas of treatment.

This is not a statement about pornography or penis enlargement – good or bad – but a simple observation that men are easily tempted in this direction. It is certainly enticing for any man to think that a way to solve his PD problem is to get a larger penis. Any man would love to think this is true, and that is exactly what the porno and penis enlargement folks want the desperate reader to think.

What man does not have the desire for a larger penis lurking in the back of his head anyway, even without having PD? But to gently suggest that a larger penis will make the penis straighter, harder or remove the lumps, is to play into the tender emotions and hopes of all men with PD. It is not fair, it is not correct, and it is a danger that a man will waste time, money and effort in that direction when there are so many other things that he really should be doing that actually make sense.

The people who direct the porn and penis enlargement sites know that most men will eventually submit to the temptation sooner or later, and will enter the site looking for sexual stimulation. This is probably a good business move for the porn and penis enlargement people, but it does not help the guy with PD even one little bit.

Here is an interesting observation about the penis enlargement sites: After a person is lured into the site by a title like, "CURE YOUR PEYRONIE'S," or he stumbles into one accidentally, PD is never mentioned again – nothing – nor is there ever an explanation of how enlarging the penis will actually help PD. It is as if they know that once you enter their site you will quickly forget your interest in PD and focus instead on their products and pornography.

The desire to have a penis that is larger than the one you were given is not recent, although it does have some current cultural basis. Men have been using dangerous methods of penis enlargement for thousands of years. Perhaps our current interest in penis size comes from various popular news and information sources concerning what women are supposed to prefer. Perhaps from eons long ago, when we all ran around naked and the size of each male organ in the tribe was well known to everyone, a large penis was associated with virility and power. Just as many attitudes and feelings are said to be genetically programmed into our brains, there might be a genetic inclination to want a larger penis.

Logically, a larger penis does not make a difference in procreation, but based on the staggering number of Internet sites that offer dozens of strategies and promises for a bigger penis, the desire must be universal and very powerful.

- ### *Effectiveness of Enlargement Products*

   No real and verifiable proof has ever been shown that any of these products actually produce a penis that is permanently larger. Read the reports and discussions from men who have used these various devices and you find they have had to spend a tremendous amount of time, hours, ever day over many months, working to achieve just a 1-2 inch temporary increase in size.

   Yet, the position taken by **PDI** is not a direct condemnation of the various techniques or devices used to increase penis size, or whether these products work or not, or even the actual value of a decision that someone makes about wanting a larger penis in the first place.

144

The **PDI** position is that if you did indeed create a larger penis by whatever method you chose, it would still have PD, and the PD would probably be worse because of the technique you used to stretch out the tissue of your penis – you would have a larger penis with a greater PD problem. This is a safe and logical conclusion, based on the reality of the hundreds of men who have reported from their own sad personal experience with these devices.

Most men I have talked to in this area concede that they would be happy and most grateful to get their old penis back in a healthy and normal state, and they are not really interested in increasing the size of anything at the moment.

Most women I have talked to in this area seem to have very little interest or fantasy about a larger penis. Those women who have to deal with a man who actually has a truly large penis often complain about the real life problems of dealing with one.

It all seems to come down to another one of those male fantasies.

• *Another Danger of Penis Enlargement*

Another potential danger is found in essentially all of the "male enhancement" gimmicks that are found all over the Internet. Any mechanical device that is intended to enlarge the size of the penis by any means of forceful stretching has the potential to do damage to the penis, with only limited benefit at most. The problem with any device that stretches the soft tissue of the penis is that no one can determine ahead of time when to stop. Depending on the individual technique, equipment used, and how aggressively it is applied, no one can safely determine when the stretching should stop. It is easy to overdo the procedure, since it is impossible to know how much is too much — **until it is too late, and further injury is caused.**

When used as the only method of treatment – as it is presented in most of these sites – it is not a good idea since simple stretching of scar tissue is insufficient to cause reversal. From our experience at **PDI** we find that all therapies work better when coupled together with many others – this is called synergy.

Even if it were possible to perform penis stretching gently and correctly, without damage to the delicate tissues, and it was effective in making the penis permanently larger – if everything worked out the way it is supposed to work, but usually doesn't – you would have a larger penis that still has a PD scar contained within. Not only that, but it would still have problems of curvature and loss of ability to become erect. Nothing of importance or therapeutic benefit would actually happen to your PD, and you would have taken a grave risk to accomplish nothing.

145

But what would probably happen, as it has in all cases of which I am aware, is that something would go wrong. Every man to whom I have spoken reports that he overused the device and hurt himself. These comments come from men who are angry with themselves because they either started their PD by overzealous stretching, or made their PD worse in the same way. The most significant flaw in the application of any stretching or enlargement method is that most men can be counted on to overuse and abuse the stretching technique. Men are just that way, it seems. If a little is good, a lot must be better. Once the process is started and some success is achieved, most men will simply apply too much force, for too long, and eventually hurt themselves. This is supported by evidence from men who have done so, time and again.

Over the years I have spoken to many, many men whose PD started because of using these very same devices that are being promoted as beneficial for PD. These men are often angry for hurting themselves in their foolish desire for a larger penis. These same men are so sorry that they deliberately did something so damaging because of a trivial and unproven goal.

• *Dangerous Enlargement Methods and Devices*

Jelqing – A penis stretching technique from ancient Persia, used for thousands of years, and still practiced in Iraq, Iran, and other Middle Eastern counties. Jelqing is a common practice in those cultures that are severely male dominated; those that place a strong emphasis on "manliness" and so take inordinate pride in a large penis.

This technique for penis enlargement involves the use of strong and sustained stretching of the penile tissue by "milking" blood from the base of the penis, up and toward the head or glans. This can be thought of as similar to squeezing a balloon at one end to expand the other end. This over-inflation of the penis is an attempt to forcefully increase the length and width by repeated stretching of the internal tissue with more blood than normally collects in the organ.

To be most successful, the force must be prolonged and heavy or the tissue will not become stretched sufficiently for the size changes that a man might be looking to achieve. If you think that the body cannot be distorted by prolonged stretching forces, just think of the over-sized lips and earlobes that are prized in some African tribes. I have spoken to many men who so traumatized themselves with the severe stretching jelqing method in particular that they developed PD from it. Probably more than any other, jelqing is the technique most often mentioned as the cause of tissue damage and eventual PD.

Just as an aside, for those who might consider that the idea of a larger penis is worth the potential risks involved, please recall the pictures you have seen of the people of the Amazon and African regions who ritually stretch their necks, ear lobes and lips as a way of becoming more attractive in their cultures. Yet, this distortion does not look very attractive to anyone I know.

These changes take years to achieve, but they are only temporary in the sense that the rings and discs that are used must be kept in place or all progress is lost. In addition, the body part that is so distorted is not healthy and functional as it was before being stretched. The necks of these women are not strong, they do not turn in a useful or normal fashion, and they are prone to many degenerative changes.

Think of that in terms of a larger penis. Perhaps you might be able to temporarily increase the length and diameter, but it is probably more prone to circulatory problems and inability to maintain the erect state.

VED – Vacuum Erection Device – This is generally a plastic cylinder fitted with an air pump at one end, and open at the other end that can be placed over the relaxed or flaccid penis. An air tight seal is created at the open end of the VED, using a water-soluble gel or lubricant like K-Y. The penis is placed inside the open end of the cylinder, and held firmly against the skin where the penis is attached to the lower abdomen. The air pump is used to draw air out of the cylinder in which the penis has been placed; the vacuum effect inside the cylinder causes a negative pressure response inside the penis. Because of the vacuum that is created, a greater than average amount of blood is drawn into the penis. What results is a larger erection than normal, the size of which is determined by how strong the vacuum force is created within the cylinder.

During this time the penis is engorged with more blood than average, and the cavernous tissues of the penis are stretched by the negative atmosphere inside the cylinder.

The extreme dilation of all penile tissues causes a dull ache and fullness that is proportionately related to the degree of negative pressure exerted on the tissue. This discomfort can increase greatly to the point of marked pain and numbness of the penis if taken to an extreme. It is possible to break blood vessels on the surface of the penis, as well as internally, if extreme negative force is created, resulting in black and blue marks and swelling. PD can result from this trauma.

Weights – A special harness is placed on the head or glans of the penis. A weight, of variable size, is attached to the harness and is allowed to freely hang from the harness so that it pulls the penis down. In effect, the penis wears a suspended weight that stretches it.

This is perhaps a fairly direct method of stretching, but its primary flaw is that the harness must be attached so tightly to the glans or head of the penis that sores develop, almost like blisters. This is perhaps the least used method available.

Stretchers – An interesting harness and expandable frame device that also lengthens or extends the penis by traction. There are several versions of this device because of the high price attached to the technology and complexity of building such an elaborate stretching device.

In this stretcher device the head of the penis is again held in a harness, to which expandable rods are attached that can be lengthened. The other ends of the rods are attached to a ring that is placed around the base of the penis and held against the pubic area. The stretcher device is so made that a sustained and controlled traction force is created by making the rods longer and longer over time, in an attempt to slowly stretch the penis.

As with the weights on the glans harness, many men I have spoken to report they cannot tolerate the soreness that develops from the friction and pressure to the delicate tissue of the penis.

- ### *About Penis Enlargement in General*

It seems as though every man I have ever spoken to about his experience with penis enlargement reports that he was not able to control his enthusiasm and excitement when he saw his penis larger than he had ever seen it before.

Many men report feeling like a kid in a candy store; they just got carried away and forgot to use good judgment. In a desire to become more "manly looking," each got injured by doing too much, too soon. For some, who saw the potential danger, or who simply could not use the device because of pain and bruised tissue, their injury was only temporary. For others, who endured the pain caused by the excessive force, they often permanently damaged internal penile tissues. The end result was the beginning of PD.

Normal tissue of the penis is not the same as the scar tissue and will not respond the same when stretched; these are dissimilar tissues and will not stretch at the same rate or degree. So if you actually could stretch the tissue of the penis that has PD, normal cavernous tissue would stretch at one rate and degree while the scar would stretch much less. This would definitely result in an even greater curvature problem. Like the slogan says, "Don't fool with Mother Nature."

It is difficult to understand how these very expensive products can be advertised as a possible treatment for PD, when they often cause PD. There are significant ethical and moral problems in such a contradiction. It is difficult to understand how these people can sleep at night.

It Is Dangerous to Underestimate Your Enemy

Very often as I talk to a man for the first time about how he wishes to start treating his PD with Alternative Medicine therapies, he will say something like, "Oh, I don't know what I really want to do. Maybe I shouldn't even bother doing anything about it right now. My problem isn't really all that bad; I mean, all I have is just one little bump and the bend I have hasn't prevented me from having sex like we always have done. I just thought maybe I should do something about it because I read these horror stories that some men tell."

This common attitude is understandable. If a man's problem is small, if it is a manageable situation, if it isn't really slowing him down much, what's the big deal anyway? Why make a big fuss if you are one of the lucky ones with a mild case of PD?

The answer is simple: A small case of PD doesn't always stay small.

Many men relate how after a year or two of living with a mild case of PD in which they had fairly good erections, no pain, minimal curvature, they woke up one day with a monster of a problem between their legs! Sudden worsening of the bend, greater pain, bottle neck, corkscrew or cane-handle deformities, and impotency, can all appear rather quickly in cases that were previously mild for a long time. This sudden worsening can happen without additional sexual injury or any known reason for the worsening. Yes, it does happen. No one can predict with reasonable certainty what will or will not happen to you. A doctor can recite certain statistics and probabilities, and give you a "Las Vegas estimate" of what will happen with your particular case, but it all comes down to this being an educated guess – nothing more than a guess. With so much at stake, it seems foolish to take that kind of chance.

In another section of this book, "Helpful Advice to Follow" in Chapter 7, we discuss many strategies that a man can follow to prevent further injury to his penis, and thus avoid subsequent worsening of his PD. When armed with some ideas to protect what you have, you will go a long way to keep that small problem small, or at least do what you can to keep your problem from getting drastically out of control.

At least a few times a day I advise someone that all cases of PD should be treated aggressively, no matter how minor they might appear at the time.

It is far better to treat a small case to keep it that way, so that it is less likely to become a major unmanageable problem later. If your problem is not all that extensive or limiting, be grateful but do not underestimate how the situation can change against you.

Potential Danger Lurks in All Sexual Situations

A high percent of men with PD report they can trace the start of their problem back to a specifically painful and traumatic event that took place during intercourse, or during masturbation with some type of mechanical device. In addition, medical texts recognize that for the man with PD, most sexual activity, especially sexual intercourse with the female partner in the superior position, carries a greater risk for direct injury to the penis than other intercourse positions. For this reason, the "female superior" intercourse posture should always be considered a strong potential danger to your penis. Don't avoid it, just be very slow and cautious when you enjoy it.

The entire subject of sexual intercourse – in all its wonderful complexity and range of possibilities – cannot be adequately considered in this book. For this reason I have written a second book, "Peyronie's Disease and Sex," that addresses the many details of sexual problems that PD couples encounter, and their possible solutions. You can go to the Peyronie's Sex Education web site at http://www.peyronies-sex-education.com/sex-and-peyronies-disease.html for further details about this book.

Potential Danger Lurks in Medications

A number of drugs list Peyronie's disease as a possible side effect. Most of these drugs belong to a class of blood pressure and heart medications called "beta blockers." One beta blocker is an eye drop preparation used to treat glaucoma, but most are used for cardiovascular and hypertension problems.

Other drugs that may cause Peyronie's disease are interferon, which is used to treat multiple sclerosis, and Dilantin, an anti-seizure medicine. The chances of developing Peyronie's disease from any of these medicines are not great, however. Any patient should check with their doctor before discontinuing any prescribed drug.

If you have PD and are taking any of these medications, please contact the doctor who prescribed it to you.

Potential Danger Lurks in the Surgical Treatment of PD

A good surgeon will only consider the more aggressive treatment of surgery for Peyronie's disease if a patient has a sufficiently severe problem to justify the risk. All surgeons are keenly aware of the frequency of poor surgical outcomes, no matter how skillful the surgeon. These unfortunate outcomes are a fact of life that are used to influence the decision for or against surgery.

In making that decision, a surgeon will guide a patient through a process that is based on many factors that describe each PD case. This is the same process that is used for most any health problem for which surgery is an option:

1. **Severity of the condition**. This is perhaps the most important factor that is evaluated in deciding about any surgery. Only when PD seriously limits sexual function is it worth the risks and rewards – and expense – of surgery.

2. **Time and opportunity for normal healing have passed**. At least 12 months from the start of PD should have lapsed for all possible healing and repair to occur. When a condition has not healed or repaired on its own, there comes a point at which the surgeon will determine that it is better to intervene.

3. **Non-response to other therapy**. During the 12 months wait a man can use a variety of drug and natural therapies to assist healing. Usually, in standard medical thinking, drugs are the first line of active treatment, but when they fail the second – surgical – line of treatment is then used.

4. **Stability**. Surgical outcomes are best for men whose condition has not improved or worsened for a while. This can be a variable time period, even in PD. Based on the other factors of the case it can be a few months to a year or more.

Peyronie's Disease Surgery Overview

Usually, Peyronie's disease surgery is performed on an outpatient basis under general anesthesia, and the procedure can last up to two and a half hours. A second doctor, a plastic surgeon, may be needed when specialized grafting techniques are used. Surgery for Peyronie's disease is a major event to a very sensitive part of the body that has a large nerve supply, so do not expect an easy walk in the park.

The degree of distortion and plaque development in the soft tissue of the penis, as well as location and general health of the individual determine the surgical technique that is used in each case. These multiple factors determine the specific outcome that is expected, and should be explained by the surgeon on a case to case basis.

Risks of Peyronie's Disease Surgery

Martin K. Gelbard, MD, states, "Unfortunately, surgery does not offer a cure for Peyronie's disease. The scarring in men with deformity severe and persistent enough to warrant an operation represents an irreversible loss of connective tissue elasticity. Though surgical restoration of sexual function can be both effective and reliable, potential candidates need to understand the compromise inherent in this approach." Compromise means that after surgery some degree of the original curvature problem and sexual limitation usually remains, and new problems can occur in spite of the best effort of the Peyronie's disease surgeon.

It comes down to this: The PD surgery might make you 25% better, or it might make you 25% worse. Approximately half of PD surgeries do not result in any change – except for the scars and the additional loss of length and girth that always remain. These are not good odds. With so little reward, these risks are difficult to justify. Those who consider undergoing surgery often do not want to hear about this common aspect of surgical outcomes, or never think that a bad outcome could happen to them.

The fact is medical texts clearly state that every surgical procedure has risk; none are totally safe or foolproof. Peyronie's disease surgery does not restore the penis to its former condition. The men I have spoken to about their PD surgery have all reported that they never really thought surgical results could be as disappointing as each had experienced – reduced penis length by 1-2 inches, scaring, new bends, pain, greater erectile dysfunction than prior to surgery due to permanent surgical alteration of blood flow in the penis, loss of penile rigidity (hardness) or inability to maintain an erection (impotence), less straightening of the penile curvature than promised, tendency toward excess scar formation, and rejection of surgical implants that requires additional surgery.

It should be of considerable concern that the Nesbit technique, one of the more popular PD procedures being used today, as described below, clearly boasts about its 50-60% success rate. While this success rate might truly be higher than average for PD surgeries, the fact is ignored that a 50-60% success rate can also be called a 40-50% failure rate. These are not very encouraging odds to all except the most desperate of men – and surgeons.

Peyronie's Disease Surgery Options:

- **Nesbit Plication** This technique or one of several variations involves gathering or pinching (plicating) tissue on the side of the penis opposite the plaque, to cause a bending force that straightens the curve. Good candidates for this procedure are those with ample penile length, and simple curvature without associated deformity (bottle-neck, hinge or hour-glass effects).

  This procedure reduces the length of the penis (1-2"), but it is not as likely to result in erectile dysfunction as other procedures such as tissue grafting; for this reason it has the highest patient satisfaction rating. Success rates of 50-60% have been reported with this technique. It is used when the bend is moderate with no loss of penile girth, and to correct a congenital curvature.

- **Tissue Grafting** This technique is the most popular removal of a Peyronie's plaque (excision). Recently, grafts have been used to expand the scar (incision).

  Excision results are disappointing with 20-70% success rates, and 16- 70% occurrence of erectile dysfunction from damage to the erectile nerves. Incision results have not yet been studied very long, although there are reports of prolonged loss of penile sensation in approximately 10% of men. Grafting is best suited for severe curves and reduced penile girth.

- **Prosthesis Implant** Small bio-compatible plastic cylinders, either solid or inflatable, are surgically inserted in the penis to make it firm. Once rather popular, implants are used less frequently since the introduction of erectile drugs (Viagra, Cialis), although they remain an option when drugs do not work.

Even with many recent improvements in PD surgical techniques, the ideal surgical procedure has not been developed. This is especially true in cases of particularly severe and complex penile curvature surgery. Recent studies of various current surgical approaches have raised concern about the long term benefits of PD surgery in relation to the risks involved.

Peyronie's disease surgery is only one option of treatment. We recommend it cautiously because, unfortunately, it can't fix everything about PD and can sometimes make a bad situation worse. For these reasons, it makes good sense that Peyronie's disease surgery should be used only as an absolute last resort after a very prolonged course of conservative therapy is applied in an aggressive manner.

In spite of these risks, there are those who should undergo surgery in an attempt to correct penile distortion and lost function, but only after solid long-term efforts with Alternative Medicine therapies have been unsuccessful in making the problems of PD more livable. **PDI** is not against the use of surgery, but it does take a strong position against using surgery before more conservative measures have been exhausted.

Final Thoughts on Limiting the Dangers Associated with PD

In spite of PD, or any other health problem, a man still has to live. He must still be able to do things, enjoy life, and feel good about himself. Yet, he should be very cautious about doing things that are risky and foolhardy for his health and well-being. We have discussed at some length those situations, habits, activities and products which pose a significant risk to the delicate tissue of the penis. Now that you have been forewarned with information and ideas about these dangers to you PD scar, you can protect yourself and avoid further deterioration. PD is a lousy problem; don't take any chances.

Chapter 11 – What to Do If Not Responding to Treatment

Ω - **To live a better life, be happier and healthier in spite of your PD, and increase your chance of successfully treating it …**

… you must know how to handle your own therapy in all its phases. No one else cares as much about your success as you do, and no one ultimately knows as much about your unique case of PD. (Actually, ALL cases of PD are unique – that is the problem.) It is going to be necessary to manage your therapy and respond to the good and bad developments that occur as you attempt to cure your own PD. This chapter will help you to understand how to approach the good and bad times.

One of the hallmarks of PD is that it usually follows a wildly variable course from one person to the next, or even from one day to the next – this is what makes PD so difficult to scientifically study and research.

You will probably not respond in your PD therapy plan like anyone else, because that is the nature of PD. With this in mind, it is necessary that you have reasonable expectations and be patient with yourself as you set out to treat this disease that has been called "the doctor's nightmare."

Attitude Problems That Will Work against You

Here are some possibilities why you might not experience the same results as someone else:

1. **Not enough treatment time**. How much time someone else needed to get results has nothing to do with you. You might need more time, and you might need less. You should begin your treatment of PD with a long-term horizon. Realize that you are making an investment of time, energy and money into getting well. Few people fail to get results if they are patient enough to invest enough effort in their recovery.

   Everyone knows how fast you gain weight or lose weight will be different from other people, and how much or how little sleep you need is different from other people.

   Yet, you are setting yourself up for disappointment, frustration and perhaps defeat, if you make the mistake of comparing yourself to others who achieved faster results. When you start comparing results with others and creating a sense of expectation in yourself that is based on the experiences of others, you create a serious problem for yourself. It is easy to understand why people compare and expect certain tings to happen, but it is also easy to understand why this measurement and comparison is inherently counterproductive. Remember, one of the hallmarks of PD is that it is such a unique and variable condition; this is the exact reason that it has defied scientific study – it is so variable in all aspects. Having said that, it is no surprise that each person will follow his own unique path of recovery. By measuring success or failure on a time-table that is based on someone else's recovery is unfair to everyone.

Most men are so eager for improvement with their PD that they create unreasonable hopes and expectations for themselves that will only harm them in the long run.

There are a few men who achieve quick and surprising degrees of improvement with their PD – sometimes in less than a month. But there are so many more men who experience only slow and irregular progress – sometimes taking six months, or longer, to see any progress whatsoever.

When I am answering email questions about therapy plans that seem to be getting no results, I always ask about how the scar and curve are being monitored.

If someone has not taken the time to measure, evaluate, and document his problem carefully, or is very careless and casual about these things, he is setting himself up for failure. It is extremely difficult to be confident that progress is happening when the starting point has not been well documented. Please go to Chapter 4, "Evaluate Your PD Scar like a Scientist."

2. **Not following your plan faithfully**. You must be consistent and aggressive in your treatment.

   If you try to learn to play the piano by faithfully practicing twice a month, you will never get anywhere.

   You cannot accomplish something as difficult or important as recovering from your PD if it is a "sometimes effort." You must be as stubborn as your PD, and as dedicated to your own success as if your life depended on it.

   Often I will advise a man to become wrapped up in treating his PD. He should have the freedom to become obsessed with following his plan and getting well. He should approach his treatment plan with the same enthusiasm and energy he puts into fishing or golfing on his day off. Think of treating your PD as a great hobby that will pay wonderful dividends. Read and learn as much as you can about it, get involved with it, spend time and energy on it, spend money on it, get wrapped up in it, just like anything else that is important to you.

3. **Not doing enough; your plan is too small.** Please go over the information in the **PDI** web site under the heading "Treatment Options," and then "Introduction."

If you try to get stronger and develop muscles by lifting weights only when you feel like it, you are doomed to be the skinniest guy on the beach.

What you put into something is usually what you can expect to get out of it. There are many laws that govern the Universe dealing with work and energy. It all comes down to the harder you work the more you get.

One of the guiding principles of treating PD is the use of the synergy.

Synergy (sin'-er-gee) is the interaction of two or more substances or forces that when combined tends to produce a total effect that is greater than the sum of the individual elements.

A short explanation of synergy is "1 + 1 +1 = 5." Taber's medical dictionary defines it as "the harmonious action of two agents such as drugs, or organs such as muscles, producing an effect which neither alone could produce, or an effect that may result which is greater than the total effects of each agent operating by itself." Synergy is neither good nor bad; it is just the compounding or growth of effects and results that occur when a group of forces are united. In other words, three bad little boys can produce a lot more trouble and chaos when working together, than they could if they were kept apart. And, conversely, three good little boys can produce a lot more good and beneficial results when working together, than they could if they were kept apart. You might think of synergy as the "teamwork effect."

Here is a very good example of synergy in everyday life. A doctor must closely monitor the combined effects of drugs that are prescribed to a patient. The effect of drug A on the body might be well known, and the effect of drug B might also be well known. But the synergistic effect of combining drugs A and B can be difficult to predict. As a result the doctor must closely monitor a patient when multiple medications are being administered. Thus, synergy is a significant part of the art of medicine.

PDI's treatment philosophy makes a lot of sense when you think about taking advantage of the power of synergy. We are suggesting that you take advantage of a simple and frequently seen phenomenon that occurs all around us every day, just as in other applications commonly seen in medical practice, architecture, agriculture, or any other part of life. The synergistic effect applies in countless areas and situations, and the treatment of PD is no different. Therefore, the synergy of multiple therapies selected from successful PD research and studies should result in an improved ability of the body to heal and repair itself.

Most people would be surprised to hear some of the conversations I have with men who go about treating their PD as if they were being asked to do a favor for an enemy. They want to get rid of their PD, but only if someone can guarantee it will be quick, effortless, and economical. If that cannot be guaranteed to them, then it is too much trouble.

They are hesitant, reluctant, overly cautious, and uninvolved; they don't want to go too far into treatment least they are inconvenienced by having to remember to take a few vitamins.

Usually these men do not do well in the self-directed Alternative Medicine form of therapy.

4. **Not having reasonable expectations**. Don't expect too much too soon from your PD therapy program. Don't put unreasonable pressure and overly high expectations on yourself. All of these will immediately work against you. Try to be reasonable and fair to yourself. PD is a tough problem to begin with. Don't make matters worse by putting unreasonable pressure on yourself. Put things in perspective and just stay focused on following your plan perfectly every day.

Results will more likely develop if you are positive and persistent.

A baby takes about nine months to develop. A young mother can really want to see her baby, but God and the baby don't care, it will still take all the time it needs to get the job done.

A farmer plants seeds one day and then goes fishing for a while. He can want to get his crops out sooner, but he knows that is not the way it works.

Ever look in at a seed catalog and notice that some tomato seeds grow and mature in 110 days, while others take 90 days or 120 days? Time is built right into the process. Get used to it.

Nature will have her way. Each process of nature is more complex and susceptible to intervention by influences and circumstances than we can ever understand. Be patient.

Variable Progress

Many men have followed the **PDI** treatment plan and obtained quick results, sometimes noticeable change in just a week or two – but they are the exception, the great exception, not the rule. We have worked with many men who have seen improvement in their PD – even after having it for many years – even after their surgeon said the only way out was by surgery – even after the problem had been declared stable and incapable of change or improvement – even after all other therapies failed – even after the distortion and pain were considered terrible. But almost all of them required time to achieve their improvement.

Usually, progress comes to men who are the "heavy hitters", treating their PD aggressively and with passion. When I speak to them I can hear determination and resolve in their voice. They throw themselves into the project of healing and recovery, and they are enthusiastic. These men who succeed are patient, single-minded, and do not allow themselves the luxury of being discouraged. They set their mind on a goal and that is all they focus on. As one of my favorite clients said once, "Hey, this is my only penis. I gotta do all I can to get it back."

Perhaps if you do not feel that same level of enthusiasm and conviction it is because you have not taken the time to educate yourself about the Alternative Medicine therapy process, and the kind of good science that is behind it. Perhaps you have just started thinking about taking control of your problem, and you are not convinced that it is possible to strengthen and support your ability to heal your own PD scar.

Just bear in mind the idea is fairly simple – perhaps too simple:

1. PD heals in 50% of the cases.

2. Alternative Medicine therapies are used in aggressive combination to assist the healing process to develop the well-known reaction called "synergy" in which the total is greater than the sum of the individual efforts.

3. Alternative Medicine therapies used by **PDI** all have some proven – although limited and sporadic – success against PD.

4. **PDI** Alternative Medicine therapy program consists of these broad categories of treatment:

    • Aggressive vitamin, mineral and enzyme supplements

    • Diet modification

    • Kegel isometric exercise

    • Deep tissue massage to increase blood and lymph flow

    • Energy medicine concepts

5. Progress with PD is measured in small steps that must be studied closely; these are often variable (good days, followed by bad days, followed by good and bad, over and over again) with a slow and steady trend of improvement over time.

6. It is better to do something, than wait around, feeling and behaving like a PD victim. You might be surprised by what your body can do when given half a chance.

"But I Have Been At It for Three Weeks Now, and Nothing Is Happening!"

Here is something to consider: Be very careful of the method(s) you are using to gauge your progress, or lack of progress. Are you sure you are being careful enough when you check yourself out that you actually will notice small changes when they occur?

If you have heavy calluses on your fingers and you work so hard with your hands that you do not have a highly sensitive touch, perhaps you are not in a good position to judge and evaluate your own progress.

In that case, my friend, ask her to help you! What a great thing for a guy to be able to ask: "Honey, would you mind coming over here and check out my penis?" Get her involved, you know she wouldn't mind helping you. At the same time you can hope that more will come of it than a simple evaluation and measurement. Make a game of it. Keep that spark of life and love going.

She needs the attention and compliment that come from you wanting her to touch you again in a sexual way. You need the attention and comfort that she wants to touch you again in a sexual way. This is a good way to make it happen. Get playful again. Use this as a great way to reconnect on a sexual level. Don't let PD beat you up and take everything away from you. It could be the beginning of a nice way to get reacquainted with your spouse.

In PD, you are attempting to measure and evaluate progress of something that is rather difficult to "put a handle on." If you are not being as careful and exact as you possibly can be, then it is certainly possible to not notice the real changes that are going on. It would be a shame if you did not notice your small but significant improvement in the early phase of self-treatment, simply because you were not looking for the subtle differences that were right there to be discovered by a knowing touch.

Please go to Chapter 5, "Monitor Your PD Scar," and reread the information about evaluating your problem. You want to be able to do a really great job of seeing the good things that are happening that you might be missing, as well as avoid the mistake of wanting and wishing for progress so badly that you fool yourself into seeing progress that is not there. Knowing the exact condition of the scar and bend is a very important step in recovery. Please pay attention.

You have to be patient with yourself, my friend. Everyone wants to get well fast – especially with this problem. That's part of society today – immediate gratification, impatience if you have to wait, and a sense of urgency in all that we do. Put things in perspective and think about the changes that you are attempting to make in yourself. Healing and repair takes time, and depending on the unique circumstances of your situation you will perhaps follow a course like no one else.

"What Can I Do Now to Get Better?"

Everyone gets discouraged early in PD treatment. For some men a surprising – shocking – response to lack of improvement is to do less to help themselves when their current effort is not getting immediate results. Can you imagine?

Imagine a young Arnold Schwarzenegger looking in the mirror one day and saying, "Gee, I don't look very muscular today, and I don't really feel very strong either. I am getting discouraged with all this bodybuilding work. Wait, I know what I will do. I think I'll exercise less. Yes, that's it. Things are not going the way I want, so I'll just do less of everything." Imagine someone in a sinking ship thinking, "The ship is sinking even thought I am bailing water, maybe I should just slow down or stop bailing water. Maybe that will improve my situation."

Arnold and any good sailor never came to those conclusions. But that is basically what I read all the time in emails from all over the world. "This is too difficult. I have been taking the vitamins for six weeks now and nothing is happening. I'll just stop for a while and see what happens." What logic! You know exactly what will happen – nothing! And, of course, the man who uses this logic fails to understand that he is setting himself up for self-induced failure.

If no wind blowing on a day when you want to fly a kite, and you really want to fly it anyway, then you just have to get busy and run like crazy to make your own wind. You can "get it up," excuse the pun, but it will just take some extra effort.

To push your progress along faster, I would suggest that you go over the **PDI** web site and consider adding one or two different products to your PD therapy program. You might want to consider also using some of the external therapies. Many men make the mistake of only loading up on the vitamin E and the systemic enzymes, but do not do much to bring energy into their body with the great external therapies that are available.

There is always something more a person can do to improve the situation. Sometimes the answer is rather obvious. We often don't see it because we are looking for something easy, and not for something that works.

160

Conclusion

The overriding mission of this book has been to assist the reader to understand his Peyronie's disease problem better than he ever has before; to gain a mastery of his situation so he no longer feels like an uninformed and confused victim of this wretched disease; and to improve the therapeutic results of his Alternative Medicine therapy. If all of this is achieved than it should follow that he will be able to lead a healthier, happier, more normal and more productive life.

If any of the expressions and phrases used in this book give the impression that improvement and mastery over PD can be guaranteed or that it is an easy or rapid accomplishment, then I have failed to adequately express the true case. Progress will almost always be slow, and irregular; sometimes, for reasons described many times throughout this text, no progress or improvement occurs at all. Some days in which the scar and the curvature show definite progress are often followed by bad days in which all previous problems return: progress, and regression, progress, and regression, back and forth. Just like the stock market: up and down and up and down and up and down, again. But over time – if your notes and records are clear and detailed – you should slowly start to see that the good days soon are more numerous than the bad days. The progress lasts longer and is clearer, while the regression becomes milder and more rare. Slowly progress takes hold and does not lose ground to regression, and you slowly allow yourself to gain confidence and excitement about what you are witnessing. It is truly a great feeling to know that you are not doomed to the life of a celibate freak.

If you are not sure of what you have read here, and if you believe from what you have read in other places that you are going to carry this secret problem with you for the rest of your life, then that is unfortunate. If that is the way you assess your problem, then I only ask that you take what appeals to you out this discussion of the many therapeutic possibilities available to you, and give it a fair and decent effort. If you cheat on what you do and how you do it, you only cheat yourself. Be fair to yourself, and be fair to her. Give it a good effort, because from what I can see – and I have looked this terrain over very well – this is the only logical and reasonable therapeutic direction that is available to you in all the world for this lousy problem called Peyronie's disease.

Even though PD is a discouraging and frustrating tragedy, do not allow yourself to give in to the fatal luxury of despair and pessimism. PD is a stubborn disease, but do not allow it to be more stubborn and determined than you are. PD is a miserable secret that is more common than anyone knows. Do not allow that to keep you from achieving your own level of success – whatever that may be – and regain your dignity and self-satisfaction as a man.

Peyronie's Disease is an extraordinary health problem and it requires an extraordinary level of effort, commitment and determination to conquer it. If you don't believe this, look around you and notice all the men who have failed. Please do your best to not be one of them.

Good luck and be successful in all that you do!

161